The Lost Bible of Natural Herbal Remedies
Time-Tested Encyclopedia Featuring 100+ Ancient Healing Recipes
for Holistic Health and Well-Being

Copyright 2025 by Evelyn Sagewood

The Lost Bible of NATURAL HERBAL REMEDIES

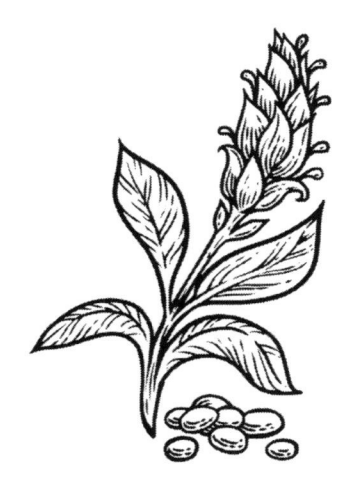

Time-Tested Encyclopedia Featuring 100+ Ancient Healing Recipes for Holistic Health and Well-Being

EVELYN SAGEWOOD

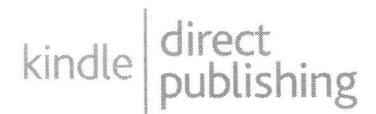

kindle direct publishing

Table of Contents

Chapter 1: The Origins of Ancient Herbal Remedies 10

    The History of Herbal Medicine 11

    The Philosophy of Natural Healing 13

    How Ancient Remedies Address Modern Health Problems 15

    Integrating Time-Tested Practices into Today's Lifestyle 17

    The Science Behind Herbal Efficacy 20

Chapter 2: Boosting Immunity Naturally 24

    Understanding the Immune System 25

    Top 5 Herbal Recipes to Strengthen Immunity 27

        1. Elderberry Immune Elixir 28

        2. Echinacea Herbal Tea 30

        3. Garlic and Honey Tonic 32

        4. Turmeric Golden Milk 34

        5. Astragalus Immune Soup 36

Chapter 3: Enhancing Digestive Health 38

    Common Digestive Issues and Their Causes 39

    Top 5 Herbal Recipes for Digestive Wellness 41

        1. Peppermint Soothing Tea 42

        2. Ginger Digestive Aid 44

        3. Fennel Seed Chewables 46

        4. Chamomile Relaxation Infusion 48

        5. Dandelion Detox Salad 50

6. Table of Contents

Chapter 4: Relieving Stress and Anxiety 52

    The Impact of Stress on Overall Health 53

    Top 5 Herbal Recipes for Calm and Relaxation 57

        1.   Lavender Relaxation Tea 58

        2.   Ashwagandha Stress Relief Tonic 60

        3.   Valerian Root Sleep Aid 62

        4.   Passionflower Calming Infusion 64

        5.   Lemon Balm Serenity Syrup 66

Chapter 5: Supporting Respiratory Health 68

    Understanding Respiratory Ailments 69

    Top 5 Herbal Recipes for Respiratory Support 73

        1.   Eucalyptus Steam Inhalation 74

        2.   Mullein Lung Tea 76

        3.   Thyme Cough Syrup 78

        4.   Licorice Root Respiratory Tonic 80

        5.   Peppermint Chest Balm 82

Chapter 6: Promoting Cardiovascular Wellness 84

    The Importance of Heart Health 85

    Top 5 Herbal Recipes for a Healthy Heart 89

        1.   Hawthorn Berry Heart Tonic 90

        2.   Garlic and Olive Oil Spread 92

        3.   Ginkgo Biloba Circulation Tea 94

        4.   Motherwort Heart Support 96

        5.   Turmeric Anti-Inflammatory Latte 98

Chapter 7: Nurturing Skin Health 100

    Common Skin Conditions and Natural Solutions 101

    Top 5 Herbal Recipes for Radiant Skin 105

        1. Aloe Vera Healing Gel 106

        2. Calendula Skin Salve 108

        3. *Tea Tree Acne Spot Treatment* 110

        4. Rose Water Facial Toner 112

        5. Oatmeal and Honey Exfoliant 114

Chapter 8: Improving Sleep Quality 116

    Understanding Sleep Disorders 117

    Top 5 Herbal Recipes for Restful Sleep 121

        1. Valerian Root Sleep Tea 122

        2. Hops Sleep Pillow Sachet 124

        3. Magnolia Bark Nighttime Tonic 126

        4. California Poppy Relaxation Elixir 128

        5. Chamomile and Lavender Bedtime Tea 130

Chapter 9: Natural Pain Management 132

    Causes of Chronic and Acute Pain 133

    Top 5 Herbal Recipes for Pain Relief 137

        1. White Willow Bark Tea 138

        2. Turmeric and Ginger Anti-Inflammatory Shot 140

        3. Arnica Muscle Rub 142

        4. St. John's Wort Oil 144

        5. Devil's Claw Pain Tonic 146

8. Table of Contents

Bonus Chapter 10: The Top 10 Healing Plants - Detailed Profiles 148
   Introduction to Nature's Most Powerful Healers 149
      1. Echinacea 150
      2. Turmeric 152
      3. Ginger 154
      4. Garlic 156
      5. Lavender 158
      6. Chamomile 160
      7. Aloe Vera 162
      8. Ginseng 164
      9. Peppermint 166
      10. Calendula 168

Conclusion 171
Regards 172

Chapter 1

The Origins of Ancient Herbal Remedies

- The History of Herbal Medicine
- The Philosophy of Natural Healing
- How Ancient Remedies Address Modern Health Problems
- Integrating Time-Tested Practices into Today's Lifestyle
- The Science Behind Herbal Efficacy

The History of Herbal Medicine

The history of herbal medicine is a rich and complex narrative that stretches back thousands of years, intertwining with the development of human civilization itself.

Long before the advent of modern pharmaceuticals, people relied on the plants around them for healing, nourishment, and spiritual guidance.

Our ancestors, through trial and error, discovered that certain herbs could relieve pain, soothe wounds, and improve overall well-being. Over time, this knowledge was passed down through generations, becoming the foundation of traditional healing practices across the world.

One of the earliest records of herbal medicine comes from ancient Mesopotamia, around 2600 BCE, where clay tablets inscribed with lists of medicinal plants were discovered. These early texts indicate a sophisticated understanding of plant-based remedies. The Sumerians, Babylonians, and later the Assyrians all employed herbs such as myrrh, fennel, and thyme for medicinal purposes. Similarly, the ancient Egyptians created detailed texts like the "Ebers Papyrus," written around 1550 BCE, which catalogued hundreds of plant-based treatments, including the use of aloe vera, garlic, and juniper.

In ancient China, herbal medicine became a cornerstone of Traditional Chinese Medicine (TCM). Dating back to at least 2000 BCE, Chinese herbal medicine was systematized with works like the "Shen Nong Ben Cao Jing" (Divine Farmer's Materia Medica), attributed to the mythical figure Shen Nong, who is said to have tasted hundreds of herbs to classify their properties. The Chinese developed a sophisticated approach to herbal medicine, balancing the yin and yang energies of the body and promoting harmony through the use of herbs such as ginseng, ginger, and licorice. These treatments were often prescribed in complex formulas tailored to each individual.

Across the Indian subcontinent, Ayurveda emerged as a comprehensive medical system, with roots dating back over 3,000 years. This ancient practice, outlined in sacred texts like the "Charaka Samhita" and "Sushruta Samhita," emphasized the use of herbs such as turmeric, ashwagandha, and neem to restore balance between the body's doshas – Vata, Pitta, and Kapha. Ayurveda remains a vibrant tradition today, reflecting an unbroken lineage of herbal wisdom.

In ancient Greece and Rome, figures like Hippocrates, often called the "father of modern medicine," and Dioscorides contributed significantly to the Western understanding of herbal medicine. Hippocrates advocated for the use of herbs in treating various ailments, promoting a holistic approach to health, while Dioscorides' "De Materia Medica" (circa 50-70 CE) became one of the most influential herbal texts in history. This five-volume work described hundreds of plants and their medicinal uses, many of which – such as willow bark (the precursor to aspirin) – are still recognized today.

Medieval Europe saw the continuation of herbal traditions through the work of monastic orders, particularly in the monasteries where monks cultivated herb gardens and copied ancient manuscripts. Hildegard of Bingen, a 12th-century Benedictine abbess, was one such figure who compiled her own herbal compendium, blending Christian spirituality with natural medicine. The rise of apothecaries during this period further cemented the role of herbal medicine in everyday life, as herbalists and healers provided remedies for common ailments.

12. Ch. 1 - The Origins of Ancient Herbal Remedies

The knowledge of indigenous peoples around the world also represents a vital chapter in the history of herbal medicine. In the Americas, Native American tribes utilized a wide array of local plants for healing. The Cherokee, for example, used black cohosh and goldenseal for women's health and wound care, while South American shamans prepared powerful concoctions from the rainforests' vast botanical resources. These traditions continue to influence contemporary herbal practices.

With the dawn of the Renaissance in Europe, herbal medicine gained new momentum. Scientific inquiry flourished, and botanists like Nicholas Culpeper compiled extensive herbal guides that merged empirical observation with traditional knowledge. Culpeper's "The Complete Herbal," published in 1653, became a household reference for herbalists and laypeople alike, promoting the medicinal virtues of plants such as lavender, dandelion, and chamomile.

The Industrial Revolution and the subsequent rise of modern medicine in the 19th and 20th centuries brought about a shift in how society viewed health and healing. Synthetic drugs, developed from active compounds originally found in plants, largely replaced herbal remedies in mainstream medicine. Despite this, many cultures retained their herbal traditions, and the resurgence of interest in natural remedies in the late 20th century marked a return to these ancient practices.

Today, herbal medicine continues to play a significant role in healthcare around the world. It is often integrated with modern medical treatments to create complementary and alternative therapies. As scientific research continues to validate the efficacy of many traditional herbal remedies, herbal medicine is being increasingly recognized as a legitimate and valuable part of holistic health.

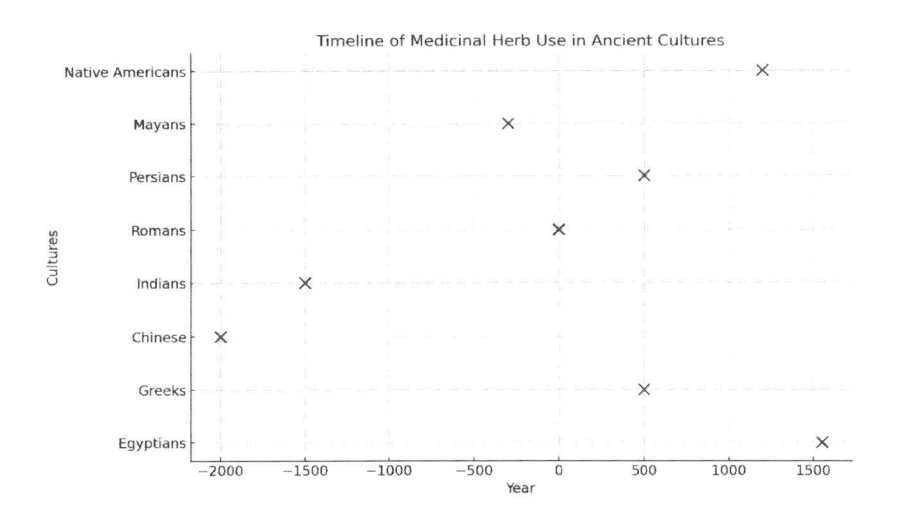

Here is a timeline chart that shows when different ancient cultures began using medicinal herbs. Each point represents a culture, such as the Egyptians, Greeks, Chinese, and others, and the approximate time period when they introduced specific herbal practices.

The Philosophy of Natural Healing

The philosophy of natural healing is grounded in the belief that the body possesses an inherent ability to heal itself, given the right conditions. This principle, often referred to as the "vital force" or "innate intelligence," emphasizes the body's natural processes of regeneration and self-repair. Natural healing seeks to support and enhance these processes rather than suppress symptoms, which is often the approach of conventional medicine. At its core, this philosophy embraces the idea that true health is more than the absence of disease – it is a state of balance and harmony, not only within the body but also between the individual and their environment.

One of the central tenets of natural healing is the concept of *holism*, which recognizes that the body, mind, and spirit are interconnected. Rather than focusing on isolated symptoms or individual body parts, holistic healing aims to treat the whole person. This philosophy encourages individuals to look at all aspects of their lives – physical health, emotional well-being, diet, lifestyle, and even their relationships with others and the natural world – as contributing factors to overall health. The idea is that by addressing imbalances in one area, the entire system can be brought back into equilibrium.

Natural healing also stresses the importance of prevention. The philosophy advocates for proactive measures to maintain health, such as proper nutrition, regular physical activity, adequate rest, and stress management. These preventive strategies are designed to strengthen the body's defenses, making it less susceptible to illness in the first place. This contrasts with conventional medicine, which often intervenes only after symptoms appear.

A fundamental aspect of natural healing is the use of *natural remedies* – plants, herbs, minerals, and other substances derived from the earth. These natural therapies are chosen for their gentleness and their ability to work in harmony with the body's biological systems. For thousands of years, cultures across the world have relied on these remedies to treat a wide range of conditions. The philosophy behind using herbs or other natural substances is that they are more aligned with the body's chemistry than synthetic drugs, which may have unwanted side effects or cause imbalances in other systems.

In the philosophy of natural healing, the individual is encouraged to take an active role in their own health. Rather than being a passive recipient of medical treatment, the patient is seen as a participant in the healing process. This empowerment is central to many natural healing traditions, as it fosters a deeper understanding of one's body and its needs. The relationship between practitioner and patient is often more collaborative than in conventional medicine, with the practitioner guiding the patient toward greater self-awareness and healthier choices.

Diet and nutrition are also vital elements in the philosophy of natural healing. Food is considered a form of medicine, and what we eat is seen as having a profound impact on our health. A nutrient-dense diet, rich in whole foods, fresh vegetables, fruits, and herbs, is thought to nourish the body on a cellular level, providing the essential building blocks for repair and vitality. The emphasis is on consuming natural, unprocessed foods that retain their full spectrum of vitamins, minerals, and enzymes, all of which are believed to contribute to the body's healing potential.

The philosophy also embraces the concept of balance, particularly in terms of how one interacts with nature and the environment. Many natural healing systems, such as Traditional Chinese Medicine (TCM) and Ayurveda, stress the importance of aligning one's lifestyle with the cycles of

Ch. 1 - The Origins of Ancient Herbal Remedies

nature – eating seasonally, adjusting daily routines to match natural rhythms, and being mindful of the energetic balance between the body and its surroundings. This alignment is believed to promote harmony, which in turn supports physical, emotional, and spiritual health.

Natural healing also places significant value on the role of the mind and emotions in health. The philosophy acknowledges that mental and emotional states can deeply influence physical health, often manifesting as symptoms in the body. Practices such as meditation, mindfulness, and stress reduction techniques are integrated into many natural healing systems to foster mental clarity, emotional resilience, and a peaceful state of mind. It is widely believed that a calm and centered mind can lead to improved physical health and a greater capacity for healing.

Another key element of natural healing is *personalized care*. Since every individual is unique, with different constitutions, lifestyle factors, and health challenges, there is no one-size-fits-all approach. Natural healing takes into account these personal differences, aiming to provide treatments that are tailored to the specific needs of the individual. Whether through herbal remedies, dietary changes, or lifestyle adjustments, the goal is to create a personalized healing plan that supports the body's natural capacity to thrive.

In its essence, the philosophy of natural healing is one of *respect for the body* and its wisdom. It encourages a shift away from the idea that health can be restored solely through external interventions, and instead, promotes the view that healing is an internal process, one that can be nurtured through thoughtful care, natural remedies, and lifestyle choices that align with nature's principles. It asks individuals to listen to their bodies, trust in their natural rhythms, and make choices that foster long-term well-being.

Ultimately, the philosophy of natural healing is about fostering a deep connection with nature, recognizing that we are not separate from the world around us, but rather a part of a larger ecosystem. By living in harmony with the natural world, using its resources wisely, and honoring the body's own intelligence, natural healing offers a path to sustainable health and wellness that goes beyond mere symptom management. It invites us to embrace a fuller understanding of health – one that honors both our bodies and the world we inhabit.

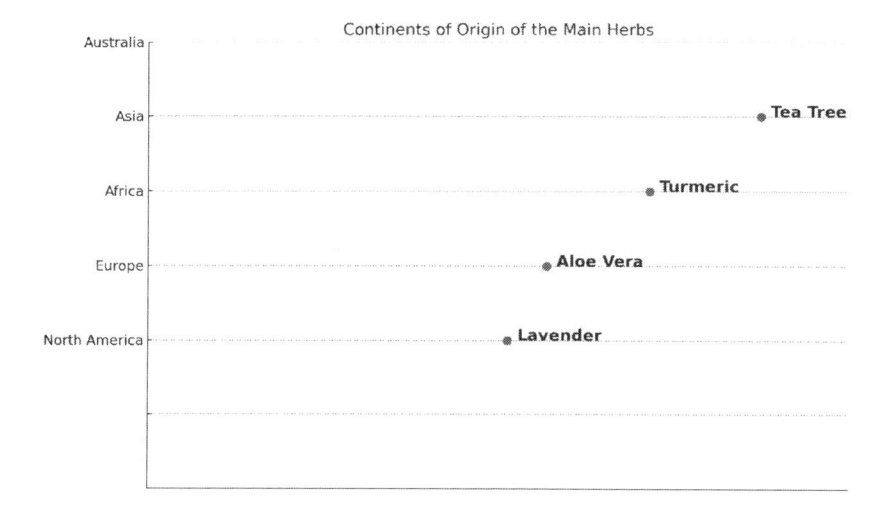

Continents of Origin of the Main Herbs

Continent	Herb
Australia	
Asia	Tea Tree
Africa	Turmeric
Europe	Aloe Vera
North America	Lavender

Here is a simplified map showing the continents of origin for key medicinal herbs.

How Ancient Remedies Address Modern Health Problems

Ancient remedies, rooted in the wisdom of traditional herbal medicine, have gained renewed attention in addressing modern health problems. As people seek alternatives to pharmaceutical treatments and strive for holistic approaches to wellness, these time-honored remedies offer valuable insights into managing both chronic and acute conditions prevalent in today's world. The resurgence of interest in ancient healing traditions – whether from Ayurveda, Traditional Chinese Medicine (TCM), Native American practices, or Western herbalism – reflects their continued relevance and effectiveness in tackling issues such as stress, inflammation, digestive problems, and immune system disorders.

One of the most significant contributions of ancient remedies to modern health is their ability to manage *chronic stress*. In today's fast-paced world, stress-related conditions such as anxiety, insomnia, and burnout are more prevalent than ever. Traditional systems like Ayurveda and TCM have long recognized the impact of emotional and mental well-being on physical health. Adaptogenic herbs – such as *ashwagandha* from Ayurveda or *ginseng* from TCM – are increasingly studied for their ability to help the body adapt to stress, reduce cortisol levels, and promote emotional resilience. These herbs, used for centuries, are known to restore balance in the body by modulating the stress response without overstimulation, unlike some modern medications.

Similarly, ancient remedies offer natural solutions to the epidemic of *inflammation* that underlies many chronic conditions today, such as heart disease, arthritis, and autoimmune disorders. Anti-inflammatory herbs like *turmeric*, rich in curcumin, have been used in Indian and Southeast Asian traditions for thousands of years. Modern science now recognizes turmeric's powerful anti-inflammatory properties, which are comparable to, and in some cases more sustainable than, synthetic drugs like NSAIDs, but without the same gastrointestinal side effects. *Boswellia* (frankincense), another ancient remedy, has also been rediscovered for its ability to reduce inflammation, particularly in the joints, making it valuable for arthritis management.

Digestive health, another area of concern in modern life, can also benefit from ancient remedies. With the rise of processed foods, sedentary lifestyles, and stress, digestive disorders such as irritable bowel syndrome (IBS), acid reflux, and bloating have become commonplace. Ancient systems of medicine have long emphasized the importance of digestion in overall health. Herbs such as *ginger*, *peppermint*, and *fennel* have been used for millennia to soothe the digestive tract, reduce gas and bloating, and enhance nutrient absorption. Ginger, in particular, is a staple in both Ayurvedic and Chinese medicine for its ability to ease nausea and improve digestion. These remedies work by promoting the healthy function of the digestive system, addressing the root causes of discomfort rather than merely masking symptoms.

The rise in autoimmune diseases and compromised immune systems in modern society has also led to a renewed focus on ancient herbal remedies known for their *immune-boosting* properties. Medicinal mushrooms, such as *reishi*, *shiitake*, and *chaga*, have been used in traditional Chinese and Japanese medicine for centuries. These mushrooms are rich in beta-glucans, compounds that help modulate the immune response, enhancing the body's ability to fight off infections while preventing excessive immune reactions, which can lead to autoimmune flare-ups. Another ancient herb, *echinacea*, used by Native American tribes, has seen a resurgence as a popular remedy for boosting the immune system, particularly in warding off colds and respiratory infections.

16. Ch. 1 - The Origins of Ancient Herbal Remedies

Ancient remedies also provide natural solutions to the growing problem of *antibiotic resistance*. While modern antibiotics have saved countless lives, their overuse has led to the development of drug-resistant bacteria. Herbal medicine offers alternatives, such as *garlic* and *oregano oil*, which possess potent antimicrobial properties that can target harmful pathogens without contributing to resistance. Honey, particularly *Manuka honey*, was used in ancient Egypt for wound healing and has shown remarkable effectiveness in fighting resistant strains of bacteria when applied topically. These natural antimicrobials not only complement modern treatments but also provide alternatives when conventional antibiotics are no longer effective.

In the realm of *hormonal balance*, ancient remedies play a significant role in addressing modern issues such as menstrual irregularities, menopause, and thyroid dysfunction. Herbs like *black cohosh*, *vitex* (chaste tree berry), and *maca* have been traditionally used to regulate hormones, alleviate symptoms of PMS, and ease the transition through menopause. With hormonal imbalances increasingly linked to environmental toxins, stress, and lifestyle factors, these gentle, plant-based remedies offer a natural way to support the endocrine system without the need for synthetic hormone therapies, which can have undesirable side effects.

Another area where ancient remedies are proving valuable is in *cardiovascular health*. Heart disease remains the leading cause of death worldwide, driven by factors such as poor diet, stress, and lack of exercise. Ancient remedies like *hawthorn berry*, used in traditional European herbal medicine, have been shown to improve heart function, increase blood flow, and strengthen the cardiovascular system. In TCM, herbs like *danshen* (red sage) and *Chinese salvia* have long been used to support circulation and prevent blood stagnation, conditions that modern science now links to cardiovascular disease.

Finally, *mental health* challenges, such as depression and cognitive decline, are areas where ancient remedies offer promising alternatives or complementary treatments. Herbs such as *St. John's Wort*, used in traditional European medicine for centuries, have gained modern recognition for their potential in treating mild to moderate depression by increasing serotonin levels naturally. *Ginkgo biloba*, one of the oldest living tree species, has been used in Chinese medicine for millennia to enhance memory and cognitive function, and is now studied for its potential to support brain health and prevent age-related cognitive decline.

The continued relevance of ancient remedies in addressing modern health problems lies in their holistic approach. They work in harmony with the body, aiming to restore balance rather than simply suppress symptoms. While modern medicine excels in acute care and life-saving interventions, ancient remedies provide a valuable complement, offering gentler, more sustainable solutions for chronic conditions and preventive care. In many ways, these remedies serve as a bridge between ancient wisdom and modern science, reminding us that the plants and natural substances that sustained human health for millennia still hold profound healing potential in the modern world.

Integrating Time-Tested Practices into Today's Lifestyle

Integrating time-tested practices into today's fast-paced lifestyle is not only possible but can be highly rewarding, offering a path to greater well-being, balance, and health. Ancient healing traditions, such as Ayurveda, Traditional Chinese Medicine (TCM), and herbalism, offer practices that address the challenges of modern life – stress, poor diet, sedentary habits, and disconnection from nature – while fostering a deep connection with our bodies and the natural world. By adapting these long-standing methods, we can cultivate healthier routines that align with our busy schedules and still honor the wisdom of the past.

One of the most accessible ways to integrate these practices is through *mindful living*. The concept of mindfulness, deeply rooted in ancient Eastern traditions like Buddhism and Ayurveda, involves being fully present and aware of our actions, thoughts, and emotions in the moment. In today's world, where multitasking and digital distractions dominate, mindfulness offers a way to slow down and reduce stress. Simple practices such as mindful eating, where one focuses entirely on the meal, savoring each bite, can help improve digestion and promote a deeper connection with food. Similarly, incorporating short meditation sessions or breathing exercises into the daily routine – even just five minutes a day – can significantly reduce anxiety, improve focus, and restore mental clarity.

Diet is another crucial area where ancient practices can be seamlessly integrated. Both Ayurveda and TCM emphasize the importance of eating according to the seasons and one's unique body constitution, or *dosha* in Ayurveda. Today, many people struggle with processed and convenience foods that lack nutritional value and disrupt the body's natural balance. By gradually adopting a more *seasonal, whole-foods-based diet*, individuals can improve their health and energy levels. For example, eating lighter, cooling foods like cucumber and watermelon in summer, and warming, nourishing foods like soups and root vegetables in winter, supports the body's innate rhythms and promotes vitality. This seasonal approach is easy to integrate by paying attention to local, fresh produce and making small adjustments to cooking habits.

Incorporating *herbal remedies* into everyday life is another way to harness the power of ancient practices. Rather than relying solely on pharmaceuticals for every minor ailment, herbs can offer gentle, natural support for common health issues. For instance, starting the day with an *herbal tea* made from adaptogenic herbs like ashwagandha or holy basil (tulsi) can help manage stress and boost resilience, while a cup of *chamomile* or *lavender* tea in the evening can promote relaxation and better sleep. Many of these herbs are available in tincture, capsule, or tea form, making it easy to incorporate them into a daily routine. Moreover, growing a small herb garden, even on a windowsill, can create a direct connection with nature and provide fresh, medicinal herbs at your fingertips.

Movement is a key aspect of ancient wellness traditions, and integrating gentle, restorative *exercise practices* from these systems can counterbalance today's often sedentary lifestyle. Practices such as *yoga* and *tai chi*, which have roots in ancient Indian and Chinese traditions respectively, are perfect for modern times because they combine physical activity with mindfulness, breath control, and relaxation. These practices improve flexibility, strength, and circulation while calming the mind and reducing stress. Unlike intense, high-impact workouts, yoga and tai chi can be adapted to any fitness level and require very little equipment, making them easy to

Ch. 1 - The Origins of Ancient Herbal Remedies

incorporate into even the busiest of schedules. A 20-minute morning yoga routine or an evening tai chi session can make a significant difference in how one feels physically and mentally.

Another vital element from ancient healing traditions that can be integrated into modern life is *detoxification*. Many traditional systems, such as Ayurveda, emphasize regular detox practices to cleanse the body of accumulated toxins, known as *ama*. In today's world, with its environmental pollutants, processed foods, and stress, these gentle detox practices are more relevant than ever. Simple practices like starting the day with warm lemon water to stimulate digestion, using a tongue scraper (an Ayurvedic tool) to remove toxins from the tongue, or incorporating regular *fasting* periods to give the digestive system a break, are easy to integrate and can have profound health benefits. Periodic detox routines, such as a seasonal cleanse with light, easily digestible foods like kitchari (a traditional Ayurvedic dish), can also help reset the system and restore balance.

Connection with nature, a central principle in many ancient healing systems, can also be woven into modern life. The Japanese practice of *forest bathing* (shinrin-yoku), which involves spending time in nature to reduce stress and improve well-being, echoes the ancient recognition of nature's healing power. Even in urban environments, spending time in parks, growing plants, or simply walking outdoors for a few minutes each day can help reconnect us with the earth and rejuvenate both body and mind. This practice doesn't require a full retreat to the wilderness – it can be as simple as taking a mindful walk during a lunch break or tending to indoor plants, both of which help to ground and center the mind.

Finally, the ancient practice of *sleep hygiene*, which has been emphasized in various traditional systems, remains incredibly relevant today. Many people suffer from poor sleep due to modern stresses and overexposure to screens and artificial light. To integrate this ancient wisdom, individuals can adopt practices such as winding down with a calming herbal tea, using essential oils like lavender or sandalwood to relax before bed, and maintaining a regular sleep schedule. Additionally, creating a peaceful and clutter-free sleep environment, free from screens and distractions, aligns with ancient principles of promoting restful, rejuvenating sleep.

Incorporating time-tested practices into today's lifestyle does not require a drastic overhaul. By gradually introducing elements such as mindful living, herbal remedies, seasonal eating, and gentle movement, we can bring the wisdom of ancient healing systems into our modern lives. These practices, when adapted thoughtfully, can help reduce stress, improve health, and foster a deeper sense of connection with ourselves and the natural world.

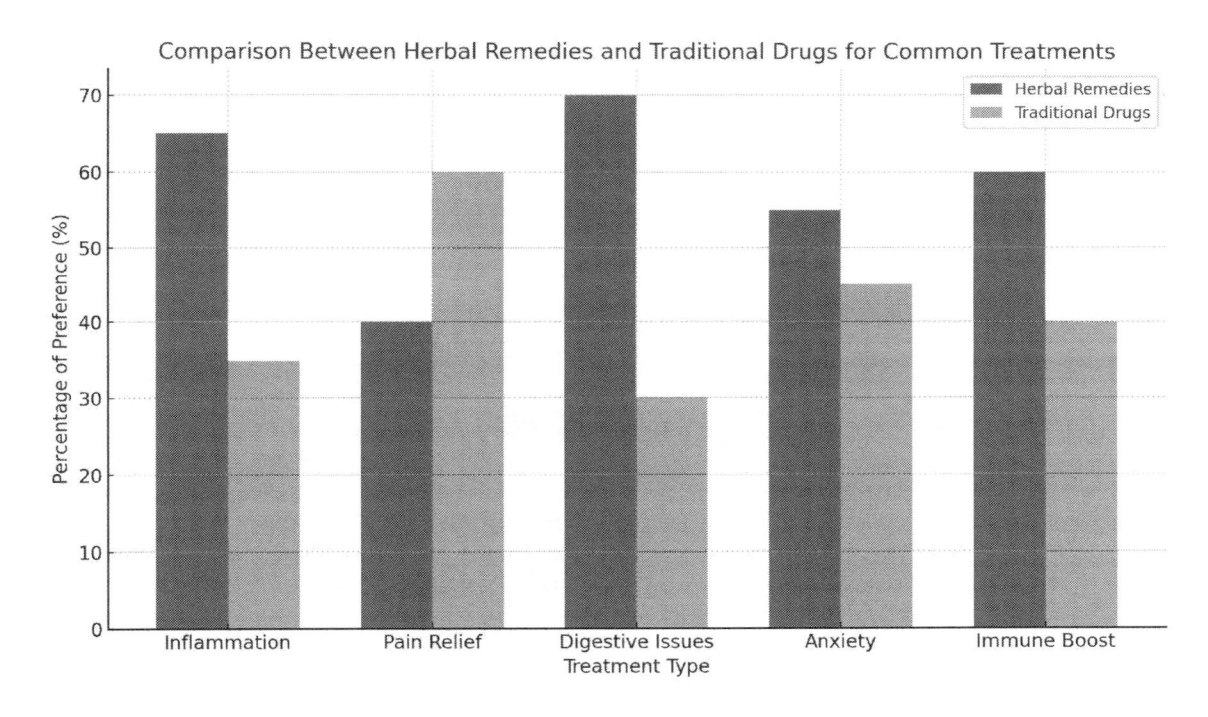

Comparison Between Herbal Remedies and Traditional Drugs for Common Treatments

Here is a bar chart comparing the use of medicinal herbs and traditional drugs for treating common issues like inflammation, pain relief, digestive problems, anxiety, and immune boosting. The chart illustrates the percentage of people who prefer herbal remedies versus those who opt for conventional medications.

The Science Behind Herbal Efficacy

The science behind herbal efficacy reveals how plants, long used in traditional medicine, have active compounds that can interact with the body in complex and beneficial ways. These compounds include alkaloids, flavonoids, terpenes, and polyphenols, among others, which have been shown to produce therapeutic effects.

Modern research increasingly supports the use of herbs for a variety of health conditions, validating many ancient practices. However, understanding how and why these plants work requires careful study of their chemical composition and the biological mechanisms they influence.

Herbs exert their effects on the body through their *bioactive compounds*, which interact with receptors, enzymes, and cells in ways similar to pharmaceutical drugs, though often in a gentler, more holistic manner. For example, the anti-inflammatory effects of *turmeric*, widely used in Ayurveda, have been attributed to its active compound *curcumin*. Curcumin works by inhibiting specific inflammatory molecules, such as NF-kB, and enzymes like COX-2, which are involved in chronic inflammation, a process linked to conditions like arthritis and heart disease. This mechanism is similar to that of synthetic anti-inflammatory drugs but without the harsh side effects often associated with pharmaceuticals.

Another herb, *willow bark*, the precursor to aspirin, contains *salicin*, a compound that the body metabolizes into salicylic acid, which reduces pain and inflammation. Ancient healers were aware of willow bark's ability to relieve pain, and modern pharmacology has since confirmed its effectiveness by isolating and synthesizing salicylic acid. While aspirin works faster and in a more concentrated form, willow bark offers similar benefits with fewer gastrointestinal side effects, highlighting how herbs can offer milder alternatives to synthetic drugs.

Herbs also play a significant role in modulating the *immune system*, and research has demonstrated how they can enhance immune response or reduce inflammation when necessary. For instance, *echinacea*, long used in Native American and European herbal medicine, has been shown to stimulate the immune system by increasing the production of white blood cells and enhancing their ability to fight off pathogens. Clinical trials have found that echinacea can reduce the duration and severity of colds and respiratory infections by boosting the body's natural defenses.

Adaptogens, a class of herbs that help the body resist stress and maintain balance, have garnered scientific attention for their impact on the body's stress response systems, particularly the *hypothalamic-pituitary-adrenal (HPA) axis*. Herbs like *ashwagandha* and *Rhodiola rosea* are now known to modulate cortisol levels and improve the body's resistance to physical, emotional, and environmental stressors. Studies on ashwagandha, for example, show that it can reduce cortisol levels, lower anxiety, and improve overall stress resilience, supporting its long-standing use in Ayurveda for managing stress and fatigue.

The efficacy of herbal medicine also lies in its ability to address *oxidative stress*, which plays a role in aging and many chronic diseases, including cardiovascular disease and cancer. Herbs rich in antioxidants, such as *green tea*, *gingko biloba*, and *rosemary*, have been studied for their ability to neutralize free radicals – unstable molecules that cause cellular damage. For example, *epigallocatechin gallate* (EGCG), a potent antioxidant found in green tea, has been linked to improved heart health, cancer prevention, and anti-aging benefits by reducing oxidative stress and inflammation in the body.

Another important aspect of herbal efficacy is their effect on *gut health*. Modern science now understands that the gut microbiome plays a crucial role in overall health, influencing everything from digestion to immune function and even mood. Herbs such as *slippery elm*, *marshmallow root*, and *licorice root*, traditionally used to soothe digestive issues, have been shown to exert their effects by creating a protective mucilage that coats and heals the lining of the digestive tract, reducing inflammation and promoting gut integrity. Additionally, many herbs act as prebiotics, providing nourishment for beneficial gut bacteria, which is essential for maintaining a healthy microbiome.

In recent years, research has also focused on the *synergistic effects* of herbs. Unlike pharmaceutical drugs, which typically involve a single active compound targeting a specific pathway, herbal remedies often contain multiple active ingredients that work together to produce a broader range of effects. This synergy can enhance the overall efficacy of the herb, as different compounds may target different mechanisms in the body or enhance the bioavailability of key ingredients.

For example, in Traditional Chinese Medicine (TCM) and Ayurveda, herbs are often prescribed in combination to create formulas that balance and enhance the effects of each plant. The classic Ayurvedic formulation *triphala*, which combines three fruits – *amalaki*, *bibhitaki*, and *haritaki* – is a well-known example of a synergistic blend that supports digestion, detoxification, and overall health.

Clinical research into herbs has also expanded, leading to randomized controlled trials and meta-analyses that provide more rigorous scientific backing for their use. For example, the herb *St. John's Wort*, traditionally used for mild to moderate depression, has been extensively studied. Clinical trials have demonstrated that St. John's Wort can be as effective as standard antidepressants like SSRIs (Selective Serotonin Reuptake Inhibitors) for treating mild depression, with fewer side effects. Its active compounds, *hypericin* and *hyperforin*, work by increasing levels of serotonin and other neurotransmitters in the brain, much like synthetic antidepressants.

However, the efficacy of herbal medicine also depends on factors such as *quality, preparation, and dosage*. Many herbs must be processed in specific ways to release their full therapeutic potential. For instance, *licorice root* can be used in its unprocessed form (Glycyrrhiza glabra) for its anti-inflammatory and antiviral effects, but when deglycyrrhizinated (DGL), it is better suited for treating gastric issues without affecting blood pressure. Standardization of herbal extracts – ensuring that each dose contains a consistent amount of active ingredients – has also been a key advancement in modern herbal science, providing more reliable results in clinical settings.

While herbal medicine is supported by increasing scientific evidence, it is important to recognize that herbs are powerful, biologically active substances. Just like pharmaceuticals, they can interact with medications or be contraindicated in certain health conditions. Therefore, the responsible use of herbal remedies, ideally under the guidance of a healthcare professional or trained herbalist, is essential to ensure safety and effectiveness.

Ch. 1 - The Origins of Ancient Herbal Remedies

In conclusion, the science behind herbal efficacy demonstrates that many ancient remedies are validated by modern research. The bioactive compounds in herbs can modulate biological pathways in ways that align with traditional uses, offering therapeutic benefits for a range of conditions. While science continues to uncover the full complexity of how herbs work, the integration of this knowledge into modern healthcare shows that plants, used responsibly, remain a potent and effective means of supporting health and well-being.

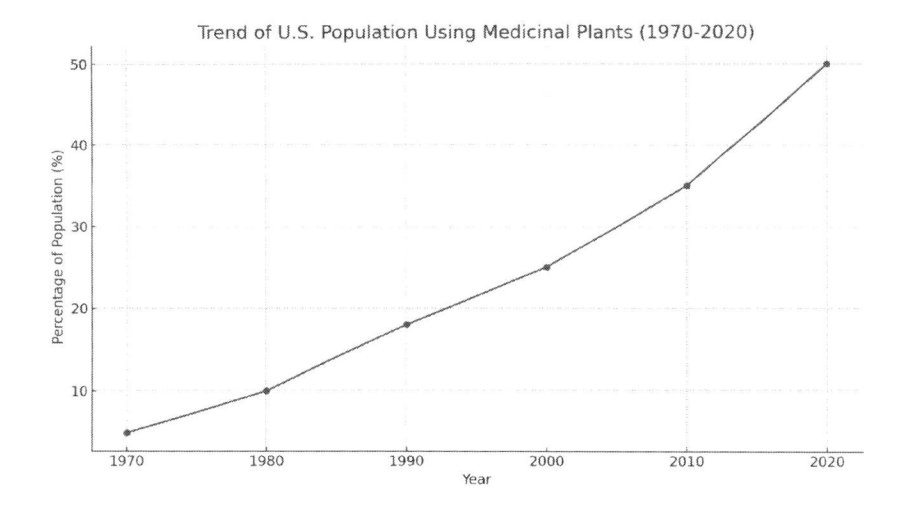

Here is the graph showing the fictional trend of the U.S. population using medicinal plants over the last 50 years (1970-2020). The graph illustrates a steady increase in the percentage of people turning to medicinal plants for health and wellness, with significant growth in the last few decades.

Chapter 2

Boosting Immunity Naturally

- Understanding the Immune System
- Top 5 Herbal Recipes to Strengthen Immunity
  1. Elderberry Immune Elixir
  2. Echinacea Herbal Tea
  3. Garlic and Honey Tonic
  4. Turmeric Golden Milk
  5. Astragalus Immune Soup

Understanding the Immune System

The immune system is a complex and dynamic network of cells, tissues, and organs that work together to protect the body from harmful invaders, such as bacteria, viruses, fungi, and toxins. Its primary role is to recognize and eliminate these foreign substances, while also distinguishing them from the body's own healthy tissues. Understanding how the immune system operates is key to maintaining health, as a well-functioning immune system is essential not only for defending against infections but also for controlling inflammation and preventing diseases like cancer and autoimmune disorders.

At its core, the immune system consists of two main components: the *innate* (or nonspecific) immune system and the *adaptive* (or specific) immune system. These two systems work in concert, with the innate immune system acting as the body's first line of defense and the adaptive immune system providing a more specialized response when the innate system is not enough to eliminate the threat.

The *innate immune system* is present from birth and provides a general defense against pathogens. It responds quickly to infections and includes physical barriers such as the skin and mucous membranes, which act as shields to block pathogens from entering the body. If pathogens manage to breach these barriers, the innate immune system uses immune cells such as *macrophages* and *neutrophils* to attack and destroy them. These cells recognize pathogens by detecting common molecular patterns found on the surface of microbes, allowing them to react swiftly but not in a highly specific way. This part of the immune system also triggers inflammation, a localized response that brings immune cells to the site of infection, helping to fight off invaders and begin the healing process.

The *adaptive immune system*, on the other hand, provides a more targeted and powerful response but takes longer to activate. It is composed of specialized white blood cells called *lymphocytes*, which include *T cells* and *B cells*. The adaptive immune system has the remarkable ability to recognize specific pathogens through receptors on the surface of these cells, and once it encounters a pathogen, it "remembers" it, offering long-term protection through *immunological memory*. This is the principle behind how vaccinations work: by exposing the immune system to a harmless version of a pathogen, the body can build up memory cells that will rapidly respond if the pathogen is encountered again in the future.

T cells play several key roles within the adaptive immune system. *Helper T cells* coordinate the immune response by signaling other immune cells, while *cytotoxic T cells* directly attack and destroy infected or cancerous cells. *B cells*, on the other hand, produce *antibodies*, which are proteins that bind to specific pathogens, marking them for destruction by other immune cells or neutralizing their ability to infect cells. Antibodies are crucial for long-term immunity, and their presence is a marker of the body's adaptive response to infections or vaccinations.

The *immune system's balance* is a delicate one, as both underactivity and overactivity can lead to health problems. When the immune system is *compromised* or weakened, as in the case of immune deficiency disorders, the body becomes more susceptible to infections. On the other hand, if the immune system is *overactive* or misdirected, it can attack the body's own tissues, leading to autoimmune diseases such as rheumatoid arthritis, lupus, and multiple sclerosis.

26. Ch. 2 - Boosting Immunity Naturally

One of the most important aspects of immune health is the ability to regulate *inflammation*. While acute inflammation is a normal and beneficial part of the immune response, chronic inflammation – where the immune system remains active and produces inflammatory chemicals over a long period – can be harmful and is linked to a variety of diseases, including heart disease, diabetes, and cancer. Keeping inflammation in check is critical for maintaining long-term health, and lifestyle factors like diet, stress management, and sleep play a crucial role in this regulation.

In recent years, research has shed light on the connection between the *gut* and the immune system, a relationship known as the *gut-immune axis*. The gut contains a large part of the immune system, with about 70-80% of the body's immune cells residing in the gut-associated lymphoid tissue (GALT). The *gut microbiome*, which consists of trillions of bacteria, fungi, and other microbes, has a profound influence on immune function. A diverse and balanced microbiome supports immune health by promoting proper immune responses and preventing overactivity. Conversely, an imbalanced microbiome, known as dysbiosis, can contribute to immune-related disorders such as allergies, autoimmune diseases, and chronic inflammation. This growing body of research emphasizes the importance of gut health for overall immune function, highlighting how diet and probiotics can modulate immune responses.

Diet and nutrition also play a fundamental role in supporting the immune system. Nutrients such as *vitamin C*, *vitamin D*, *zinc*, and *selenium* are crucial for optimal immune function. Vitamin C, for instance, enhances the production and function of white blood cells, while vitamin D is essential for activating immune defenses, particularly the response of T cells. Zinc aids in the development and function of immune cells, and selenium has powerful antioxidant properties that protect immune cells from damage. A diet rich in fruits, vegetables, whole grains, and healthy fats supports immune health by providing these essential nutrients as well as a variety of *antioxidants*, which protect against oxidative stress and support the immune system's ability to fight off infections.

In addition to diet, *lifestyle factors* such as stress management, exercise, and sleep are vital for maintaining a healthy immune system. Chronic stress can suppress immune function by raising cortisol levels, which reduces the ability of the immune system to respond to threats. Regular, moderate exercise boosts circulation, helps immune cells move more efficiently through the body, and enhances immune surveillance. Meanwhile, getting enough restorative sleep is critical for the production of cytokines, a type of protein that helps regulate immune responses. Sleep deprivation weakens the immune system, making the body more vulnerable to infections.

Top 5
Herbal Recipes
to Strengthen Immunity

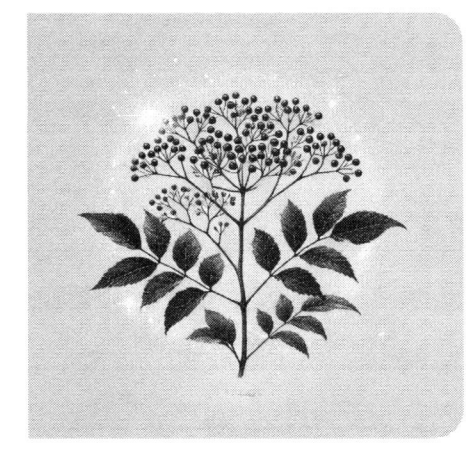

1. Elderberry Immune Elixir

An Elderberry Immune Elixir is a potent natural remedy made from elderberries (*Sambucus nigra*), known for their immune-boosting properties. For centuries, elderberries have been used in traditional medicine to ward off colds, flu, and other respiratory infections. Modern research supports their efficacy, showing that elderberries are rich in antioxidants, particularly flavonoids like anthocyanins, which help strengthen the immune system by reducing inflammation and enhancing the body's defense mechanisms. They also have antiviral properties that can help prevent the replication of viruses, particularly in the early stages of an infection.

Making an Elderberry Immune Elixir at home is both simple and rewarding, offering a natural way to support your immune system, particularly during cold and flu season. This elixir is often prepared by simmering elderberries with other beneficial ingredients, such as ginger, cinnamon, and honey, which not only enhance the flavor but also add their own therapeutic effects.

Key Ingredients and Their Benefits:

- **Elderberries**: The star of the elixir, elderberries are packed with antioxidants and vitamins A, B, and C, which help stimulate immune function. Elderberries also promote healthy circulation, reduce inflammation, and provide antiviral support by inhibiting viral entry into cells.

- **Ginger**: A well-known anti-inflammatory and antioxidant, ginger also supports the immune system by promoting circulation and aiding digestion, both of which are crucial for overall health. It has a warming effect, which can be soothing during a cold or flu.

- **Cinnamon**: This warming spice is antimicrobial and can help balance blood sugar, while also providing anti-inflammatory and antioxidant benefits. Cinnamon has traditionally been used to fight infections and promote respiratory health.

- **Honey**: Raw honey, especially if it's local or Manuka honey, has antibacterial and antiviral properties. Honey also soothes sore throats and provides a natural sweetness to the elixir, making it more palatable.

- **Cloves** (optional): Cloves are rich in antioxidants and have antibacterial, antiviral, and antifungal properties. Adding a few cloves can enhance the immune-boosting effects of the elixir while adding a rich, spicy flavor.

Basic Recipe for Elderberry Immune Elixir:

Ingredients:

- 1 cup dried elderberries
(or 2 cups fresh elderberries)

- 3 cups water

- 1 tablespoon fresh ginger root (grated)
or 1 teaspoon dried ginger powder

- 1 cinnamon stick
(or 1 teaspoon ground cinnamon)

- 1 tablespoon cloves (optional)

- ½ to 1 cup raw honey (adjust to taste)

Instructions:

1. In a medium saucepan, combine the elderberries, water, ginger, cinnamon, and cloves (if using).
2. Bring the mixture to a boil, then reduce the heat to a simmer. Allow it to simmer for 30-45 minutes, or until the liquid has reduced by about half.
3. Remove the pan from heat and let the mixture cool slightly.
4. Strain the liquid through a fine mesh strainer or cheesecloth into a clean jar or bottle, pressing down on the elderberries to extract all the juice.
5. Once the liquid has cooled to lukewarm (not hot, to preserve the honey's properties), stir in the raw honey until fully dissolved.
6. Store the elixir in a glass jar in the refrigerator for up to two weeks.

Dosage:

- **For prevention**: Take 1 tablespoon daily, especially during cold and flu season or when you're feeling run down.
- **For acute symptoms**: If you start feeling ill, take 1 tablespoon every 2-3 hours until symptoms subside.

The Science Behind Elderberry's Immune-Boosting Powers:

Several studies have demonstrated that elderberry extract can shorten the duration of colds and flu by enhancing immune response and reducing viral activity. In one study, people who took elderberry syrup saw a reduction in the severity and length of flu symptoms compared to those who did not. The flavonoids in elderberries are thought to bind to viruses, preventing them from entering and infecting healthy cells.

Moreover, elderberries are rich in *antioxidants*, which help reduce oxidative stress – a condition that can weaken the immune system and increase susceptibility to infections. By neutralizing harmful free radicals, elderberries contribute to overall immune health, making them a valuable component of this elixir.

Additional Notes:

It's important to use cooked elderberries in any remedy, as raw elderberries contain compounds that can cause nausea and digestive discomfort. Cooking the berries neutralizes these compounds, making them safe and effective for consumption.

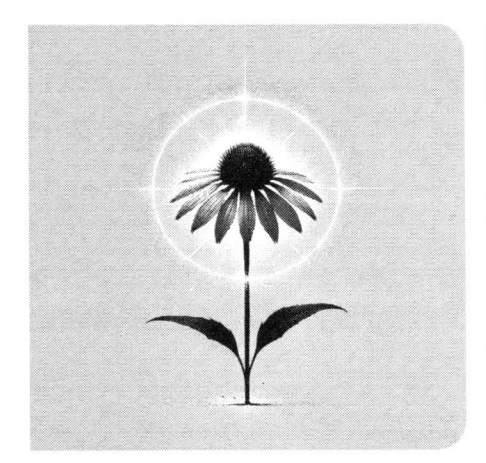

2. Echinacea Herbal Tea

Echinacea herbal tea is a popular and potent natural remedy that has been used for centuries to support immune health and fight off infections. Made from the roots, leaves, and flowers of the *Echinacea* plant, this tea is particularly valued for its ability to boost the body's immune defenses, making it a go-to remedy during cold and flu season. Echinacea, traditionally used by Native American tribes, has been scientifically studied for its antiviral, antibacterial, and anti-inflammatory properties, making it an ideal herbal tea to support overall health and resilience.

Key Benefits of Echinacea:

- **Immune-Boosting**: Echinacea is known for stimulating the production of white blood cells, which are essential for fighting infections. It activates *phagocytes* – cells that engulf and destroy pathogens – and increases the overall activity of the immune system, helping the body fend off viruses and bacteria more effectively.

- **Antiviral Properties**: Studies suggest that Echinacea can reduce the severity and duration of respiratory infections, including the common cold, by preventing viruses from replicating and spreading within the body. This makes it an excellent preventive remedy during the flu season or when exposed to viral infections.

- **Anti-Inflammatory**: Echinacea contains compounds that can reduce inflammation, which is not only important for healing infections but also for controlling symptoms like sore throat, nasal congestion, and swelling.

- **Antioxidant-Rich**: Echinacea is packed with antioxidants like flavonoids, cichoric acid, and rosmarinic acid, which help protect cells from oxidative stress. These antioxidants support overall health by neutralizing free radicals that can damage cells and compromise the immune system.

Making Echinacea Herbal Tea:

Echinacea tea is simple to prepare and can be enjoyed regularly to help strengthen the immune system or as a supportive remedy when feeling under the weather. Both fresh and dried Echinacea can be used, though dried Echinacea is more commonly available in tea form or loose herb.

Ingredients:

- 1-2 teaspoons dried Echinacea leaves, flowers, or root (or a combination)
- 1 cup boiling water
- Optional: honey, lemon, ginger, or peppermint for added flavor and benefits

Instructions:

1. Boil water and pour it over the dried Echinacea herb in a teapot or mug.

2. Cover and let the tea steep for 10-15 minutes to extract its medicinal properties.

3. Strain the tea into a cup, and if desired, add a teaspoon of honey or a slice of lemon to enhance the flavor and provide additional soothing benefits. Ginger or peppermint can also be added for extra immune and digestive support.

4. Enjoy the tea warm, sipping slowly.

Dosage:

- For **preventive** purposes, drink 1-2 cups of Echinacea tea daily, especially during times of increased exposure to colds, flu, or other infections.

- When **feeling sick**, you can increase the dosage to 3-4 cups per day to help reduce the severity and duration of symptoms.

Science Behind Echinacea's Effectiveness:

Numerous studies have explored Echinacea's role in enhancing immune function and fighting infections. Research shows that it can activate various immune cells, such as macrophages and natural killer cells, which are critical in attacking foreign pathogens. Additionally, clinical trials have demonstrated that Echinacea can reduce the risk of developing colds by about 50% and shorten the duration of cold symptoms by one to two days. Its antiviral action is linked to the ability of Echinacea's bioactive compounds, such as *echinacoside* and *alkamides*, to inhibit viral entry into healthy cells, preventing the spread of infection.

Echinacea also has anti-inflammatory effects, which can help soothe sore throats and reduce nasal congestion and swelling. These properties make it not only a preventative herb but also a useful remedy during the onset of colds or flu.

Additional Ingredients to Boost Echinacea Tea:

- **Honey**: Adding honey provides antibacterial benefits and soothes irritated throats, making it an excellent complement to Echinacea during colds.

- **Ginger**: This warming herb aids digestion and improves circulation, helping the body's immune response. It also has anti-inflammatory and antiviral properties.

- **Lemon**: Rich in vitamin C, lemon boosts the immune system further and adds a refreshing flavor.

- **Peppermint**: Adding peppermint to Echinacea tea can enhance its effects by opening up nasal passages, soothing respiratory symptoms, and aiding digestion.

Precautions and Considerations:

While Echinacea is generally considered safe for most people when used for short periods (up to a few weeks), some individuals, particularly those with autoimmune disorders or allergies to plants in the *Asteraceae* family (which includes ragweed and daisies), should consult with a healthcare provider before using Echinacea. Extended use of Echinacea, especially at high doses, may overstimulate the immune system in these cases.

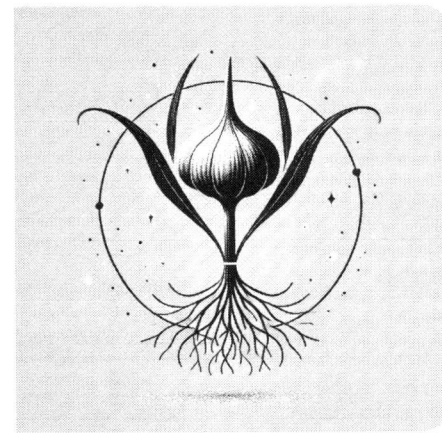

3. Garlic and Honey Tonic

Garlic and honey tonic is a powerful, time-tested natural remedy that harnesses the medicinal properties of garlic and honey to support the immune system, fight infections, and promote overall health. Garlic (*Allium sativum*) has been used for centuries as a potent antibacterial, antiviral, and anti-inflammatory agent, while raw honey is known for its soothing, antimicrobial, and antioxidant qualities. Together, these two ingredients form a dynamic combination that can help prevent and treat colds, flu, sore throats, and even digestive issues.

Key Benefits of Garlic and Honey Tonic:

- **Immune-Boosting**: Garlic contains *allicin*, a sulfur compound that is released when garlic is crushed or chopped. Allicin has strong antimicrobial properties and can help the body fend off bacteria, viruses, and fungi. Honey, particularly raw or Manuka honey, supports the immune system with its natural enzymes and antioxidants, further enhancing the tonic's ability to fight infections.

- **Antibacterial and Antiviral**: Both garlic and honey are effective in combating pathogens. Garlic's allicin disrupts the activity of harmful microbes, while honey creates a hostile environment for bacteria and viruses, making it an ideal natural remedy for respiratory infections.

- **Anti-Inflammatory**: Garlic helps reduce inflammation throughout the body by inhibiting pro-inflammatory cytokines, while honey soothes irritation, particularly in the throat and digestive tract.

- **Antioxidant-Rich**: Garlic and honey are packed with antioxidants that protect cells from oxidative stress, reducing the risk of chronic diseases and supporting overall health. Honey's antioxidants also help neutralize free radicals, promoting tissue repair and immune function.

- **Heart Health**: Garlic is well-known for its ability to lower blood pressure, reduce cholesterol levels, and improve circulation, making this tonic beneficial for cardiovascular health as well.

How to Make a Garlic and Honey Tonic:

Ingredients:
- 8-10 cloves of fresh garlic
- 1 cup raw honey (local or Manuka honey is ideal)
- A small jar with a tight-fitting lid

Instructions:

1. Peel the garlic cloves and lightly crush them with the side of a knife or chop them finely. Crushing the garlic helps release allicin, the active compound that provides many of garlic's health benefits.

2. Place the crushed garlic cloves into a clean glass jar.

3. Pour the raw honey over the garlic, ensuring that the cloves are completely submerged. Stir gently to mix the garlic and honey.

4. Seal the jar with a tight-fitting lid and let the mixture sit at room temperature for 3-5 days. During this time, the garlic will infuse its medicinal properties into the honey.

5. After 3-5 days, the tonic is ready to use. You can store it in the refrigerator, where it will continue to develop its potency and can last for several months.

How to Use:

- **For immune support**: Take 1 teaspoon of the garlic-honey tonic daily to help boost your immune system, particularly during cold and flu season.
- **For acute illness**: At the first sign of a cold or sore throat, take 1 teaspoon every few hours to help fight the infection and soothe symptoms.
- **For heart health**: Regular use of garlic and honey can help improve heart health by lowering cholesterol and blood pressure. Taking 1 teaspoon a day is beneficial for maintaining cardiovascular function.

Science Behind the Tonic:

Garlic has been extensively studied for its antimicrobial and immune-boosting effects. Allicin, the key compound in garlic, has been shown to exhibit antibacterial and antiviral properties that can help the body defend against infections. Research has demonstrated that garlic supplementation can reduce the incidence and severity of common colds by boosting the immune system's response to viruses. Additionally, garlic is known to promote heart health by lowering LDL cholesterol and blood pressure, making it a well-rounded medicinal herb.

Honey, particularly raw and Manuka varieties, contains a wealth of enzymes and antioxidants that enhance its medicinal value. Honey's natural hydrogen peroxide and methylglyoxal (found in Manuka honey) are powerful antibacterial agents that inhibit bacterial growth and speed up healing. Honey is also soothing for sore throats and coughs, making it a staple in traditional remedies for respiratory infections. Studies have shown that honey can be more effective than over-the-counter cough syrups for reducing cough frequency in children.

Variations and Additions:

- **Lemon**: Adding a few slices of lemon to the tonic enhances its vitamin C content, offering additional immune support and making the tonic even more effective at fighting colds.
- **Ginger**: Ginger can be added to the tonic for its anti-inflammatory and digestive benefits. It also provides a warming effect, which can be soothing when you're sick.
- **Cayenne Pepper**: A pinch of cayenne can stimulate circulation and provide additional antibacterial benefits, especially helpful for sinus congestion and sore throats.

Safety and Considerations:

While garlic and honey are generally safe for most people, there are a few considerations to keep in mind. Garlic can thin the blood, so individuals on blood-thinning medications or those preparing for surgery should consult a healthcare professional before using it in large amounts. Additionally, honey should not be given to children under the age of one due to the risk of botulism.

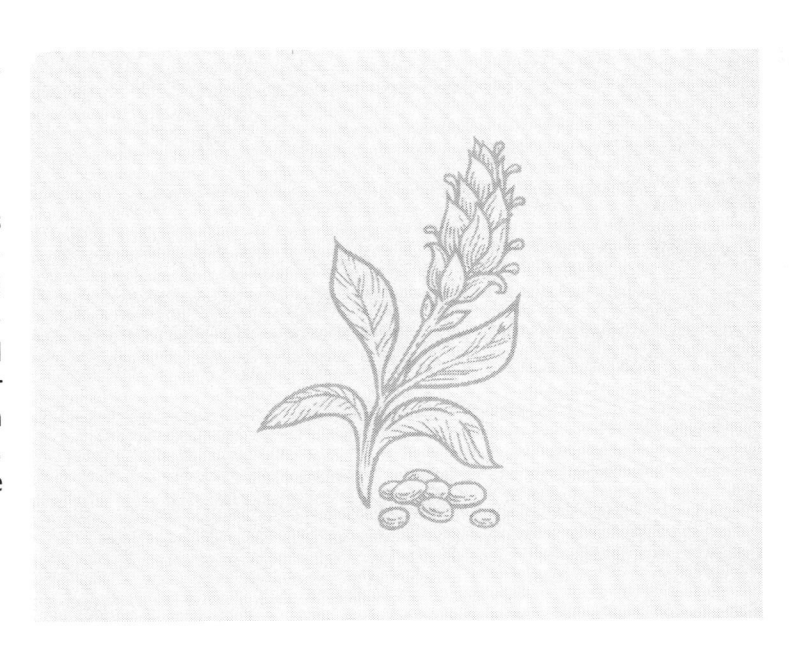

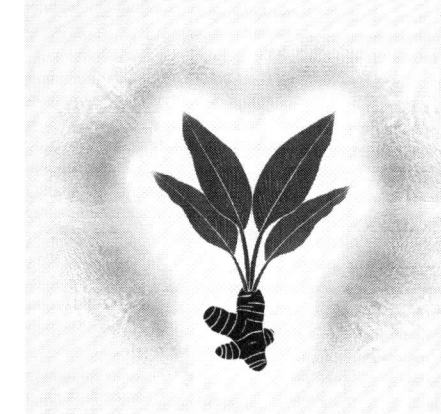

4. Turmeric Golden Milk

Turmeric Golden Milk, also known as "Haldi Doodh" in traditional Ayurvedic medicine, is a soothing and nutrient-rich beverage made from turmeric and milk, often combined with other warming spices such as ginger, cinnamon, and black pepper. This ancient remedy has been used for centuries to promote healing, reduce inflammation, and boost overall well-being. The key ingredient, turmeric, is well-known for its powerful anti-inflammatory and antioxidant properties, making Golden Milk a potent elixir for modern health challenges such as joint pain, digestive issues, and immune support.

Key Benefits of Turmeric Golden Milk:

- **Anti-Inflammatory**: Turmeric contains *curcumin*, a compound known for its ability to combat chronic inflammation. Curcumin inhibits inflammatory markers in the body, making it useful for conditions like arthritis, muscle soreness, and other inflammatory diseases.
- **Antioxidant-Rich**: The antioxidant properties of curcumin help protect cells from oxidative stress and free radical damage, which are linked to aging, cancer, and many chronic diseases.
- **Digestive Health**: Turmeric has been traditionally used to support digestion by stimulating bile production and promoting healthy gut function. It also helps reduce bloating and gas.
- **Immune Support**: Turmeric, along with other spices like ginger and cinnamon, enhances immune function by reducing inflammation and fighting infections. Ginger, in particular, has antiviral properties, and cinnamon is known for its antimicrobial effects.
- **Joint and Muscle Health**: The anti-inflammatory nature of turmeric makes Golden Milk an excellent remedy for those with joint pain or muscle stiffness, particularly in conditions like arthritis.
- **Relaxation and Sleep**: Warm Golden Milk, especially when made with a hint of cinnamon and honey, has a calming effect on the body and mind. The ritual of drinking this warm beverage before bed can promote better sleep and relaxation.

How to Make Turmeric Golden Milk:

Ingredients:

- 1 cup milk of your choice (traditional cow's milk, or plant-based alternatives like almond, coconut, or oat milk)
- 1 teaspoon turmeric powder (or 1 tablespoon freshly grated turmeric root)
- ½ teaspoon ground cinnamon
- ½ teaspoon freshly grated ginger (or ¼ teaspoon ground ginger)
- Pinch of black pepper (to enhance curcumin absorption)
- 1 teaspoon raw honey or maple syrup (optional, for sweetness)
- ½ teaspoon coconut oil or ghee (optional, for enhanced absorption of curcumin)

Instructions:

1. In a small saucepan, heat the milk over medium heat until it begins to simmer gently.

2. Add the turmeric, cinnamon, ginger, and black pepper to the milk, stirring well to combine. You can also add the coconut oil or ghee at this point to boost curcumin absorption.

3. Reduce the heat and let the mixture simmer for about 5 minutes, allowing the spices to infuse into the milk.

4. Remove from heat and strain the mixture if you used fresh ginger or turmeric root.

5. Stir in the honey or maple syrup if desired, adjusting sweetness to taste.

6. Pour into a mug and enjoy warm.

Variations of Golden Milk:

- **Vanilla Golden Milk**: Add a splash of vanilla extract for a more comforting and dessert-like flavor.
- **Spiced Golden Milk**: Enhance the warming properties by adding a pinch of cardamom, nutmeg, or even cayenne pepper for a little heat.
- **Chai-Style Golden Milk**: Combine turmeric with chai spices like cloves, star anise, and fennel seeds for a more robust and spicy version of this drink.

Science Behind Turmeric's Benefits:

Curcumin, the active compound in turmeric, has been extensively studied for its medicinal properties. Research has demonstrated that curcumin can reduce inflammation by blocking molecules such as NF-kB, which are involved in triggering the body's inflammatory response. This has broad implications for managing chronic inflammatory conditions such as arthritis, inflammatory bowel disease, and even neurodegenerative diseases like Alzheimer's.

Turmeric's antioxidant activity also protects cells from oxidative damage. Oxidative stress is a major factor in the development of chronic diseases, and curcumin helps neutralize free radicals while also boosting the body's own antioxidant defenses.

In terms of mental health, curcumin has been found to boost brain-derived neurotrophic factor (BDNF), a growth hormone that functions in the brain, which may help delay age-related brain degeneration and improve mood by reducing symptoms of depression.

Dosage and Regular Use:

For general wellness and prevention, drinking one cup of Golden Milk per day is sufficient to experience its benefits. For individuals with chronic inflammation or joint pain, consuming Golden Milk daily over an extended period may provide more noticeable relief.

Precautions:

While turmeric is generally safe for most people, high doses or long-term use can cause gastrointestinal discomfort in some individuals. It's also important for people taking blood thinners or those with gallbladder issues to consult with their healthcare provider before using turmeric regularly, as it can interact with certain medications.

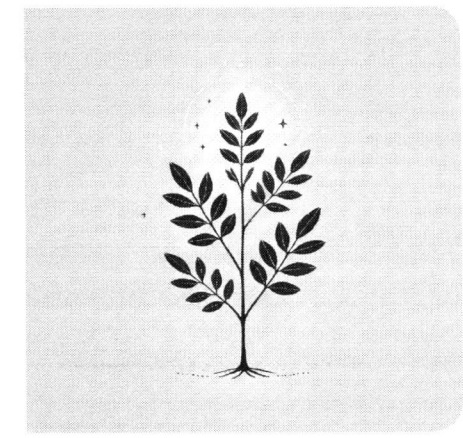

5. Astragalus Immune Soup

Astragalus Immune Soup is a nourishing and powerful herbal remedy that integrates the immune-boosting benefits of *Astragalus* root with wholesome ingredients to support overall health. Astragalus (*Astragalus membranaceus*), a staple in Traditional Chinese Medicine (TCM), is known for its ability to enhance immune function, protect against stress, and improve vitality. This herb has been used for centuries to prevent illness, particularly during the cold and flu season, by fortifying the body's defenses against infections.

Combining Astragalus with other nutrient-dense ingredients in a soup creates a comforting and healing meal that not only strengthens the immune system but also supports digestion and overall wellness. This soup is particularly helpful during times of immune stress, such as seasonal transitions or when you're feeling run down.

Key Benefits of Astragalus Immune Soup:

- **Immune-Boosting**: Astragalus is a well-known adaptogen, meaning it helps the body resist physical, mental, and environmental stress. Its immune-enhancing properties work by increasing the activity of white blood cells and promoting the production of antibodies, helping to fend off infections before they take hold.
- **Antioxidant-Rich**: Astragalus is packed with antioxidants that protect the body from oxidative stress, which can weaken the immune system and lead to chronic disease. The herb's antioxidant properties help combat free radicals and promote longevity.
- **Energy and Vitality**: In TCM, Astragalus is often used to boost "Qi" (vital energy) and improve endurance. It's an ideal herb for those who feel fatigued, weak, or depleted, as it supports the body's natural energy reserves.
- **Supports Respiratory Health**: Astragalus has traditionally been used to strengthen lung function and improve respiratory health, making it especially useful during cold and flu season when respiratory infections are common.

How to Make Astragalus Immune Soup:

This immune-boosting soup is easy to prepare and can be customized with your favorite vegetables, herbs, and proteins. The base recipe includes Astragalus root, which can be found dried in health food stores or Chinese herbal shops. Other medicinal mushrooms or immune-supporting herbs can also be added for extra benefits.

Ingredients:
- 3-4 slices of dried Astragalus root (or about 10-15 grams)
- 1 medium onion, chopped
- 3 cloves garlic, minced
- 2-3 large carrots, chopped
- 2-3 stalks celery, chopped
- 1 piece fresh ginger (about 1 inch), sliced
- 1 tablespoon olive oil (or sesame oil)
- 6-8 cups vegetable or chicken broth
- 1-2 tablespoons soy sauce or tamari (optional)
- Salt and pepper to taste
- Optional: shiitake mushrooms, leafy greens (like kale or spinach), or other vegetables of choice
- Optional: protein sources like tofu, chicken, or legumes

Instructions:

1. In a large pot, heat the olive oil over medium heat. Add the chopped onions, garlic, and ginger, and sauté for 3-5 minutes until fragrant and softened.

2. Add the chopped carrots, celery, and any other vegetables you're using, and cook for another 5 minutes, stirring occasionally.

3. Pour in the vegetable or chicken broth and add the Astragalus root slices. If you're using shiitake mushrooms or other medicinal mushrooms, add them now.

4. Bring the soup to a boil, then reduce the heat and let it simmer for 45 minutes to an hour, allowing the Astragalus and vegetables to infuse the broth with their immune-boosting properties.

5. Remove the Astragalus root slices before serving (they are tough and fibrous, so they aren't meant to be eaten). You can strain the soup if you prefer a smoother consistency, or leave it chunky for a heartier meal.

6. Season with soy sauce or tamari, salt, and pepper to taste. Add greens or protein sources during the last 10 minutes of cooking, if desired.

7. Serve warm and enjoy!

Dosage and Use:

Astragalus Immune Soup can be enjoyed as a meal throughout the week, particularly during cold and flu season or times of high stress when your immune system needs extra support. You can have it as a preventive measure, with 1-2 bowls per week to keep your defenses strong, or more frequently if you're feeling run down or recovering from an illness.

Science Behind Astragalus:

Numerous studies support the traditional use of Astragalus as an immune enhancer. The herb contains polysaccharides that have been shown to stimulate the immune system by increasing the activity of macrophages and natural killer cells, both of which are essential for fighting infections. Astragalus also promotes the production of interferon, a protein that helps the immune system respond to viral infections, making it particularly useful in preventing respiratory illnesses.

Astragalus is classified as an adaptogen, meaning it helps the body adapt to stress and maintain homeostasis. By reducing the negative effects of stress on the body, Astragalus not only strengthens the immune system but also helps prevent fatigue and improve energy levels. Studies also show that Astragalus has antiviral and anti-inflammatory effects, further boosting its reputation as a key herb for immune support.

Additional Ingredients to Boost the Soup's Benefits:

- **Shiitake Mushrooms**: These mushrooms are known for their immune-boosting properties, particularly their ability to enhance white blood cell activity. They add both nutrition and a savory depth of flavor to the soup.
- **Ginger**: Warming and anti-inflammatory, ginger aids digestion and helps the body fight infections. Its spicy, warming nature complements the immune-strengthening properties of Astragalus.
- **Garlic**: Known for its powerful antibacterial and antiviral effects, garlic boosts immune function and enhances the overall benefits of the soup.
- **Leafy Greens**: Adding nutrient-dense greens like kale or spinach provides essential vitamins and minerals, including vitamin C and iron, which further support immune health.

Precautions and Considerations:

While Astragalus is generally safe for most people when used in moderate amounts, it's important to note that it may not be suitable for individuals with autoimmune conditions, as it can stimulate the immune system. If you are on immunosuppressive medication or have a condition like lupus or rheumatoid arthritis, consult with a healthcare provider before using Astragalus regularly. Pregnant or breastfeeding women should also consult their doctor before using this herb.

Chapter 3
Enhancing Digestive Health

- Common Digestive Issues and Their Causes
- Top 5 Herbal Recipes for Digestive Wellness
  1. Peppermint Soothing Tea
  2. Ginger Digestive Aid
  3. Fennel Seed Chewables
  4. Chamomile Relaxation Infusion
  5. Dandelion Detox Salad

Ch. 3 - Enhancing Digestive Health

Common Digestive Issues and Their Causes

Common digestive issues are widespread and can significantly impact quality of life. They range from mild discomfort to chronic conditions, affecting how the digestive system processes food and absorbs nutrients. Understanding the causes of these issues is key to managing them effectively. Below, we explore some of the most common digestive problems and their underlying causes.

1. Indigestion (Dyspepsia):

Indigestion refers to a feeling of discomfort or pain in the upper abdomen, often accompanied by bloating, nausea, or a burning sensation. It can be caused by overeating, eating too quickly, or consuming fatty or spicy foods that are hard to digest. Stress and anxiety can also exacerbate indigestion by affecting the digestive system's ability to function properly.

- **Causes:** Overeating, fatty foods, alcohol, caffeine, stress, certain medications (like NSAIDs).

2. Acid Reflux (GERD):

Gastroesophageal reflux disease (GERD), commonly known as acid reflux, occurs when stomach acid flows back into the esophagus, causing a burning sensation in the chest (heartburn). This condition is often aggravated by certain foods, obesity, lying down after meals, or hiatal hernia (when part of the stomach pushes through the diaphragm).

- **Causes**: Weak lower esophageal sphincter (LES), obesity, spicy or fatty foods, caffeine, smoking, alcohol, pregnancy, and certain medications.

3. Irritable Bowel Syndrome (IBS):

IBS is a chronic condition affecting the large intestine, characterized by symptoms such as cramping, abdominal pain, bloating, gas, diarrhea, and constipation. The exact cause of IBS is unclear, but it is thought to involve a combination of factors, including abnormal gut motility, heightened sensitivity to pain in the digestive tract, food intolerances, and stress.

- **Causes**: Stress, hormonal changes, gastrointestinal infections, imbalanced gut microbiome, certain foods (e.g., dairy, gluten, caffeine).

4. Constipation:

Constipation occurs when bowel movements become infrequent or difficult to pass, often causing discomfort and bloating. It is usually the result of slow movement of stool through the digestive tract, which can be influenced by diet, lifestyle, or medication use. A diet low in fiber, dehydration, and lack of physical activity are common contributors to constipation.

- **Causes**: Low fiber diet, dehydration, lack of physical activity, certain medications (e.g., opioids, antacids), ignoring the urge to defecate, and hormonal changes (e.g., pregnancy).

5. Diarrhea:

Diarrhea involves frequent, loose, or watery stools and can be acute or chronic. Acute diarrhea is often caused by infections (bacterial, viral, or parasitic) or food poisoning, while chronic diarrhea may result from underlying conditions such as IBS, inflammatory bowel disease (IBD), or food intolerances. It can lead to dehydration and nutrient deficiencies if prolonged.

- **Causes**: Infections, food intolerances (e.g., lactose, gluten), medications (antibiotics), IBS, stress, and inflammatory bowel disease.

6. Bloating and Gas:

Bloating and excess gas are common digestive complaints often resulting from the accumulation of gas in the digestive tract. This can occur when food is not digested properly, leading to fermentation in the gut, or from swallowing air while eating. Certain foods, such as beans, lentils, broccoli, and carbonated drinks, are known to increase gas production.

- **Causes**: Swallowed air, overeating, high-fiber foods (beans, legumes), carbonated beverages, food intolerances (lactose, gluten), and imbalanced gut bacteria.

7. Peptic Ulcers:

Peptic ulcers are sores that form on the lining of the stomach or the upper part of the small intestine, often causing burning stomach pain, indigestion, and nausea. They are primarily caused by infection with *Helicobacter pylori* bacteria or long-term use of nonsteroidal anti-inflammatory drugs (NSAIDs), which damage the stomach lining.

- **Causes**: *H. pylori* infection, chronic NSAID use, excessive alcohol consumption, smoking, and stress.

8. Food Intolerances and Sensitivities:

Food intolerances occur when the digestive system is unable to properly digest certain foods, leading to symptoms such as bloating, gas, diarrhea, and stomach pain. Common intolerances include lactose (from dairy products), gluten (from wheat and related grains), and fructose (a sugar found in fruit).

- **Causes**: Enzyme deficiencies (e.g., lactase for lactose intolerance), celiac disease (autoimmune reaction to gluten), and poor absorption of certain sugars.

9. Gallstones:

Gallstones are solid deposits that form in the gallbladder, which can cause digestive issues like pain, nausea, and vomiting, especially after consuming fatty meals. Gallstones can block the bile ducts, leading to inflammation and digestive problems.

- **Causes**: High cholesterol levels in bile, obesity, rapid weight loss, pregnancy, and a diet high in fats and low in fiber.

10. Inflammatory Bowel Disease (IBD):

IBD refers to chronic inflammatory conditions of the gastrointestinal tract, the most common being Crohn's disease and ulcerative colitis. Symptoms include severe diarrhea, abdominal pain, fatigue, and weight loss. The exact cause is not fully understood, but it is believed to involve an immune response that attacks the gut lining.

- **Causes**: Autoimmune response, genetic factors, environmental triggers, smoking (especially for Crohn's disease), and infections.

Top 5 Herbal Recipes for Digestive Wellness

Ch. 3 - Top 5 Herbal Recipes for Digestive Wellness

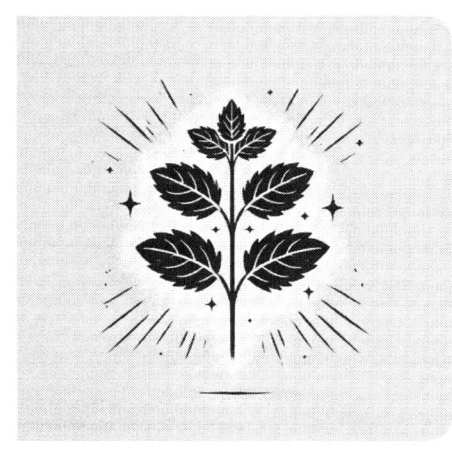

1. Peppermint Soothing Tea

Peppermint Soothing Tea is a refreshing and therapeutic herbal infusion known for its calming effects on the digestive system and its ability to relieve discomfort such as indigestion, bloating, and nausea. Made from the leaves of the *Mentha piperita* plant, peppermint tea has been used for centuries in traditional medicine for its cooling and soothing properties. The tea is rich in volatile oils, particularly *menthol*, which gives it its characteristic cooling sensation and medicinal benefits.

Key Benefits of Peppermint Soothing Tea:

- **Digestive Aid**: Peppermint tea is widely recognized for its ability to relax the muscles of the gastrointestinal tract, making it a go-to remedy for indigestion, bloating, gas, and irritable bowel syndrome (IBS). The menthol in peppermint helps reduce spasms in the gut, allowing food to pass more easily and relieving discomfort.

- **Relieves Nausea and Motion Sickness**: Peppermint has a long history of use for easing nausea and vomiting. The cooling effect of menthol can help calm the stomach, making peppermint tea an excellent natural remedy for motion sickness or morning sickness during pregnancy.

- **Antispasmodic Properties**: The antispasmodic effects of peppermint make it effective for reducing cramps and muscle spasms, whether in the digestive system or other areas of the body. This is particularly beneficial for individuals with IBS, where muscle spasms in the intestines cause discomfort.

- **Calming and Stress Relief**: Peppermint tea has mild sedative properties, making it helpful for reducing stress, calming anxiety, and promoting relaxation. Sipping a warm cup of peppermint tea can help soothe both the body and the mind.

- **Respiratory Relief**: The menthol in peppermint tea acts as a natural decongestant and can help clear the sinuses and airways, making it useful for respiratory conditions like colds, sinusitis, and allergies. Inhaling the steam from the tea can further enhance these effects.

How to Make Peppermint Soothing Tea:

Ingredients:
- 1 tablespoon fresh peppermint leaves (or 1 teaspoon dried peppermint leaves)
- 1 cup hot water
- Optional: honey or lemon for added flavor and benefits

Instructions:

1. Boil water and allow it to cool slightly (about 5 minutes after boiling).

2. Place the peppermint leaves in a teapot or mug.

3. Pour the hot water over the leaves, covering them completely.

4. Let the tea steep for 5-10 minutes, depending on how strong you prefer it.

5. Strain the tea to remove the leaves and pour it into a cup.

6. Add honey or lemon to taste if desired, and enjoy warm.

Dosage:

- **For digestive relief**: Drink 1-2 cups of peppermint tea daily, particularly after meals, to soothe the stomach and aid digestion.

- **For nausea or motion sickness**: Sip a cup of peppermint tea as needed to calm the stomach and reduce nausea.

- **For relaxation and stress relief**: Enjoy a cup in the evening or before bed to promote relaxation and help with sleep.

Science Behind Peppermint Tea's Efficacy:

The key component of peppermint's medicinal power lies in its high content of volatile oils, particularly *menthol*, *menthone*, and *limonene*. **Menthol** acts as a muscle relaxant, helping to relieve digestive issues like cramps, bloating, and discomfort. Studies have shown that peppermint oil can reduce the frequency and intensity of abdominal pain in individuals with IBS by relaxing the muscles of the gut.

Peppermint tea also has mild **analgesic (pain-relieving) properties**, making it helpful for tension headaches and minor muscle aches. Research has shown that the menthol in peppermint can act as a natural analgesic by inhibiting the sensation of pain, particularly when applied topically, but drinking peppermint tea can provide some internal relief as well.

The **antimicrobial properties** of peppermint have also been studied, showing its ability to help combat certain bacteria and viruses. This makes peppermint tea beneficial for both digestive health and respiratory conditions, as it can reduce symptoms of colds, sinus infections, and allergies by acting as a natural decongestant.

Variations and Additions:

- **Ginger**: For an extra digestive boost, add a few slices of fresh ginger to your peppermint tea. Ginger complements peppermint's antispasmodic and nausea-relieving properties and adds warmth to the tea.

- **Chamomile**: Combining peppermint with chamomile can enhance the calming and digestive benefits of the tea. Chamomile is also known for its soothing effect on the stomach and can help with sleep.

- **Lemon Balm**: Lemon balm is another calming herb that can be blended with peppermint to enhance stress relief and promote relaxation.

- **Fennel Seeds**: Add a teaspoon of fennel seeds to your peppermint tea to enhance its ability to reduce bloating and gas, as fennel is another well-known digestive aid.

Precautions:

While peppermint tea is generally safe for most people, individuals with **gastroesophageal reflux disease (GERD)** or severe acid reflux should use caution, as peppermint can relax the lower esophageal sphincter, allowing stomach acid to rise into the esophagus and potentially worsen symptoms. It is also important to avoid large amounts of peppermint tea if you are pregnant, as the menthol in high doses may cause uterine relaxation.

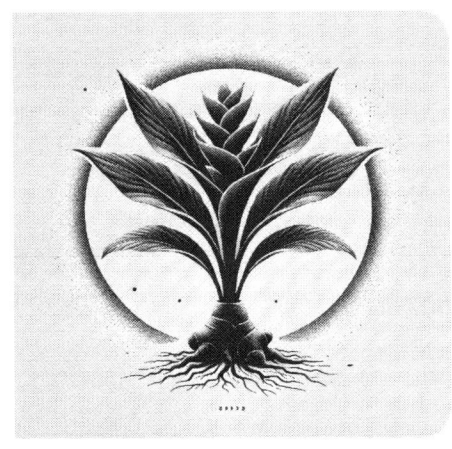

2. Ginger Digestive Aid

Ginger Digestive Aid is a natural and time-tested remedy that harnesses the medicinal properties of *Zingiber officinale* (ginger) to improve digestion and alleviate common digestive problems. Ginger has been used for thousands of years in traditional medicine systems, such as Ayurveda and Traditional Chinese Medicine, to treat nausea, indigestion, and other digestive issues. With its warming, anti-inflammatory, and carminative properties, ginger promotes healthy digestion and helps ease discomfort in the stomach and intestines.

Key Benefits of Ginger as a Digestive Aid:

- **Relieves Nausea**: Ginger is one of the most effective natural remedies for nausea, including morning sickness during pregnancy, motion sickness, and nausea associated with chemotherapy. Its active compounds, such as *gingerols* and *shogaols*, help soothe the stomach lining and prevent the brain from triggering the vomiting reflex.

- **Improves Digestion**: Ginger stimulates the production of digestive enzymes and bile, which helps break down food more efficiently, improving nutrient absorption and reducing bloating, gas, and indigestion.

- **Reduces Bloating and Gas**: As a natural carminative, ginger helps expel excess gas from the digestive tract, providing relief from bloating and abdominal discomfort.

- **Eases Indigestion and Heartburn**: Ginger can relax the smooth muscles of the intestines, allowing food to pass more easily through the digestive system and reducing the chances of indigestion and acid reflux.

- **Anti-Inflammatory**: Chronic inflammation in the digestive tract can lead to issues like gastritis, irritable bowel syndrome (IBS), or inflammatory bowel disease (IBD). Ginger's anti-inflammatory properties help soothe the gut lining, reduce inflammation, and promote healing.

How to Make a Ginger Digestive Aid (Tea):

Ingredients:

- 1-2 inches fresh ginger root, peeled and sliced (or 1 teaspoon ground ginger)
- 1 cup hot water
- Optional: 1 teaspoon raw honey or lemon juice (for added flavor and benefits)

Instructions:

1. Peel and thinly slice the fresh ginger root.
2. Bring 1 cup of water to a boil, then reduce the heat and add the ginger slices.
3. Let the ginger simmer for about 10 minutes, allowing it to steep and release its beneficial compounds.
4. Strain the ginger slices from the tea and pour the liquid into a cup.
5. Add honey or lemon juice if desired, and drink the tea warm.

Dosage:

- **For general digestive support**: Drink 1 cup of ginger tea after meals to stimulate digestion and prevent indigestion.

- **For nausea relief**: Sip on ginger tea as needed, or take small amounts of ginger (in candy or capsule form) throughout the day to relieve nausea.

Science Behind Ginger's Digestive Benefits:

Ginger's digestive benefits are primarily attributed to its bioactive compounds, particularly *gingerols* and *shogaols*, which have been shown to stimulate the production of digestive enzymes. These compounds promote efficient digestion by increasing saliva, bile, and gastric juices, which break down food more effectively and speed up the process of moving food through the digestive tract.

In several studies, ginger has been found to reduce the symptoms of indigestion (also known as dyspepsia) by improving gastric motility, meaning it helps food move through the stomach and intestines more smoothly. By enhancing gastric emptying, ginger can prevent food from lingering too long in the stomach, which is often a cause of bloating, discomfort, and acid reflux.

Research also supports ginger's effectiveness in treating nausea. A study published in the *Journal of the American Board of Family Medicine* found that ginger significantly reduced nausea and vomiting in pregnant women without adverse side effects. Similarly, ginger is widely used as a complementary treatment for chemotherapy-induced nausea, showing both its potency and safety.

Variations and Additions:

- **Ginger with Mint**: Add a few fresh mint leaves to the ginger tea for enhanced soothing of the digestive tract. Mint, like ginger, helps reduce bloating and gas.
- **Ginger with Lemon**: Add freshly squeezed lemon juice to ginger tea to increase its digestive and cleansing benefits. Lemon stimulates bile production, further supporting digestion.
- **Ginger with Fennel**: Fennel seeds are another digestive aid known for reducing gas and bloating. Add 1 teaspoon of fennel seeds to your ginger tea for extra relief from digestive discomfort.
- **Ginger and Turmeric**: Combine ginger with turmeric to create a powerful anti-inflammatory and digestive tonic. Both herbs support gut health and reduce inflammation.

Additional Benefits of Ginger:

- **Promotes Gut Health**: By reducing inflammation and promoting the secretion of digestive enzymes, ginger helps maintain a healthy gut, supporting a balanced microbiome and reducing the risk of gastrointestinal infections.
- **Boosts Circulation**: Ginger has a warming effect and helps increase circulation throughout the body, which is beneficial for digestion, as improved blood flow supports better nutrient absorption and digestive function.
- **Reduces Acid Reflux**: Unlike certain medications, ginger doesn't reduce stomach acid but rather helps it stay in the stomach by promoting healthy gastric motility, which reduces the likelihood of acid reflux.

Precautions:

While ginger is generally safe for most people, those with certain conditions, such as gallstones or ulcers, should consult a healthcare provider before using ginger regularly. Additionally, individuals taking blood-thinning medications (such as warfarin) should be cautious, as ginger can enhance the effects of these medications and increase the risk of bleeding. Pregnant women should use moderate doses of ginger to avoid potential risks.

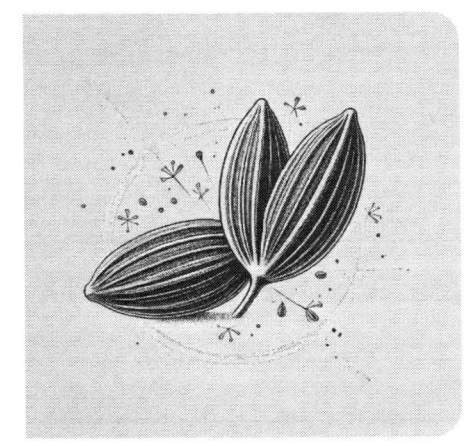

3. Fennel Seed Chewables

Fennel Seed Chewables are a simple, natural remedy used to support digestion and relieve common digestive issues such as bloating, gas, and indigestion. *Foeniculum vulgare*, or fennel, has been used in traditional medicine for centuries, particularly in Ayurvedic and Mediterranean practices, for its ability to stimulate digestion and ease discomfort in the stomach and intestines. Fennel seeds contain essential oils, including *anethole*, which have carminative, anti-inflammatory, and antimicrobial properties, making them an effective and gentle remedy for digestive relief.

Key Benefits of Fennel Seed Chewables:

- **Reduces Bloating and Gas**: Fennel seeds are known for their carminative properties, which help relax the muscles of the digestive tract and release trapped gas. Chewing fennel seeds after a meal can relieve bloating and prevent excessive gas.

- **Improves Digestion**: Fennel seeds stimulate the production of digestive enzymes and gastric juices, helping to break down food more efficiently and improving overall digestion. They are particularly useful for those who experience slow digestion or feel heavy after meals.

- **Eases Indigestion**: By promoting healthy digestion and reducing spasms in the digestive tract, fennel seeds can help alleviate indigestion and discomfort, especially after eating heavy or rich foods.

- **Freshens Breath**: Fennel seeds are naturally aromatic and have antimicrobial properties, making them effective in combating bad breath. Chewing on fennel seeds can help neutralize odors and leave your breath fresh.

- **Soothes Heartburn**: Fennel seeds can help reduce acid production and soothe inflammation in the stomach, providing relief from heartburn and acid reflux in some individuals.

How to Use Fennel Seed Chewables:

Ingredients:

- 1 teaspoon whole fennel seeds (preferably organic)

Instructions:

1. After a meal, chew 1 teaspoon of fennel seeds thoroughly. The seeds release their essential oils as you chew, which helps stimulate digestion and provide relief from bloating or gas.

2. Swallow the seeds after chewing, as they will continue to provide benefits as they pass through the digestive tract.

3. You can use fennel seed chewables after any meal, or whenever you feel digestive discomfort.

Dosage:

- **For general digestive support**: Chew 1 teaspoon of fennel seeds after meals to promote digestion and reduce bloating.

- **For bloating or indigestion**: Chew 1 teaspoon of fennel seeds at the first sign of discomfort to help ease symptoms.

Science Behind Fennel's Digestive Benefits:

The primary active compound in fennel seeds is *anethole*, which has been shown to have carminative and antispasmodic effects, meaning it helps relax the muscles of the gastrointestinal tract and prevent gas formation. Studies suggest that fennel seeds increase the secretion of digestive juices, improving the breakdown of food and reducing the risk of indigestion.

Fennel also contains *flavonoids* and *volatile oils* that have mild anti-inflammatory and antimicrobial effects. These properties help soothe the lining of the digestive tract, reduce inflammation, and combat harmful bacteria that may contribute to digestive discomfort. Additionally, fennel seeds can help normalize stomach acid production, reducing the likelihood of acid reflux and heartburn.

A study published in the *Journal of Ethnopharmacology* showed that fennel seeds significantly reduced colic symptoms and improved digestion in infants, highlighting their effectiveness in treating digestive issues in both children and adults.

Variations and Additions:

- **Fennel and Cardamom**: Combine fennel seeds with a few cardamom pods for added digestive benefits and a pleasant aromatic flavor. Cardamom is another traditional digestive aid known for relieving bloating and indigestion.

- **Fennel and Anise Seeds**: Mix fennel seeds with anise seeds for a more intense carminative effect. Both seeds share similar compounds that support digestion and reduce gas.

- **Roasted Fennel Seeds**: Lightly roast fennel seeds in a dry pan until they become fragrant, which enhances their flavor and can make them more enjoyable to chew. Roasted fennel seeds are commonly used in Indian cuisine as a digestive aid.

Additional Benefits of Fennel Seeds:

- **Helps with Appetite Control**: Fennel seeds may help regulate appetite by promoting a sense of fullness, making them useful for those looking to control overeating or manage weight.

- **Supports Hormonal Balance**: Fennel seeds contain phytoestrogens, plant compounds that mimic estrogen, which may help balance hormones and alleviate symptoms of menopause or menstrual discomfort.

- **Anti-inflammatory Properties**: The essential oils in fennel seeds have anti-inflammatory properties, which can help reduce inflammation in the gut and other parts of the body.

Precautions:

While fennel seeds are generally safe and well-tolerated, they should be used with caution by individuals with allergies to plants in the carrot or parsley family (*Apiaceae*), as fennel is part of this group. Pregnant women should also consult a healthcare provider before consuming large quantities of fennel seeds, as they contain phytoestrogens, which may affect hormonal balance.

4. Chamomile Relaxation Infusion

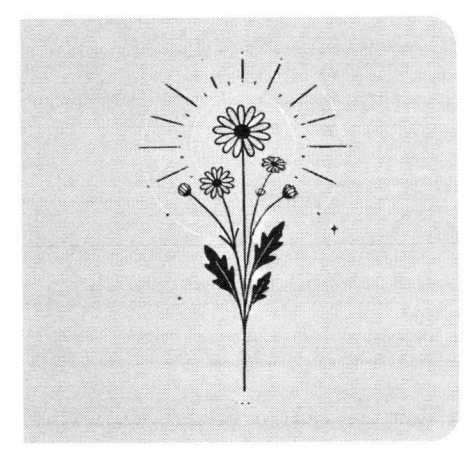

Chamomile Relaxation Infusion is a gentle, calming herbal tea made from the dried flowers of the chamomile plant (*Matricaria chamomilla* or *Chamaemelum nobile*). Known for its soothing effects, chamomile has been used for centuries to promote relaxation, reduce stress, and support restful sleep. Its natural sedative and anti-inflammatory properties make chamomile tea a perfect choice for winding down at the end of the day, easing anxiety, and relieving digestive discomforts that can interfere with rest.

Key Benefits of Chamomile Relaxation Infusion:

- **Promotes Relaxation and Sleep**: Chamomile is widely recognized for its mild sedative properties, which help reduce anxiety and tension. Drinking chamomile tea before bed can promote relaxation and improve sleep quality, making it an excellent remedy for insomnia or restlessness.
- **Eases Anxiety and Stress**: Chamomile's calming effects on the nervous system make it effective in reducing symptoms of anxiety and stress. Its gentle nature makes it a great alternative to stronger medications or supplements, particularly for those seeking a natural remedy.
- **Soothes Digestive Discomfort**: Chamomile has anti-inflammatory and antispasmodic properties that help relax the muscles of the digestive tract, making it useful for alleviating indigestion, bloating, gas, and stomach cramps. It is also helpful for reducing symptoms of irritable bowel syndrome (IBS) and other digestive disorders associated with stress.
- **Reduces Inflammation**: Chamomile contains *apigenin*, a flavonoid with anti-inflammatory properties that can help reduce inflammation in the body, soothing both internal and external discomforts.
- **Supports Immune Health**: Chamomile's antioxidant properties, particularly from its flavonoids, support the immune system by protecting cells from oxidative stress and promoting overall well-being.

How to Make Chamomile Relaxation Infusion:

Ingredients:
- 1 tablespoon dried chamomile flowers (or 1 chamomile tea bag)
- 1 cup hot water
- Optional: honey, lemon, or a few slices of fresh ginger for added flavor and benefits

Instructions:

1. Boil water and let it cool slightly for about 2-3 minutes.
2. Place the dried chamomile flowers or tea bag in a mug.
3. Pour the hot water over the chamomile, covering it completely.
4. Let the tea steep for 5-10 minutes, depending on how strong you prefer it.
5. Strain the tea (if using loose chamomile flowers), and add honey or lemon to taste, if desired.
6. Sip the tea slowly, ideally in the evening or before bed, to promote relaxation.

Dosage:

- **For relaxation and sleep**: Drink 1 cup of chamomile tea about 30 minutes before bed to support restful sleep.
- **For anxiety or stress relief**: Drink 1-2 cups of chamomile tea throughout the day as needed to ease anxiety and promote calmness.

Science Behind Chamomile's Relaxation Benefits:

Chamomile's calming effects are primarily due to its flavonoids, particularly *apigenin*, which binds to GABA receptors in the brain, similar to how anti-anxiety medications work. GABA (gamma-aminobutyric acid) is a neurotransmitter that helps reduce neuronal excitability, promoting a sense of calm and reducing feelings of anxiety. By interacting with these receptors, chamomile can help induce relaxation and improve sleep without the risk of dependency or significant side effects.

Several studies have shown chamomile to be effective in treating mild to moderate anxiety and promoting better sleep quality. For example, a study published in *Phytomedicine* found that chamomile extract significantly reduced anxiety symptoms in participants with generalized anxiety disorder (GAD) over an 8-week period.

Chamomile also contains anti-inflammatory and antioxidant compounds that help reduce inflammation in the body. This is particularly useful for soothing digestive issues like irritable bowel syndrome (IBS), indigestion, or stress-related stomach discomfort, all of which can interfere with relaxation and sleep.

Variations and Additions:

- **Chamomile and Lavender**: Combine chamomile with lavender flowers for a deeply calming tea that enhances relaxation and reduces anxiety. Lavender is also known for its sedative and soothing properties.
- **Chamomile and Mint**: Add a few fresh mint leaves to your chamomile tea for a refreshing yet calming infusion. Mint supports digestion and adds a cooling effect, making it perfect for evening relaxation.
- **Chamomile and Ginger**: For an added anti-inflammatory and digestive boost, add a few slices of fresh ginger to your chamomile tea. Ginger is warming and can help settle the stomach, especially if stress or anxiety causes digestive upset.
- **Chamomile and Lemon Balm**: Lemon balm is a calming herb that, like chamomile, helps reduce anxiety and promote restful sleep. Combining these two herbs enhances the soothing effects of the tea.

Additional Benefits of Chamomile Tea:

- **Alleviates Menstrual Pain**: Chamomile's antispasmodic properties can help relax the muscles of the uterus, reducing menstrual cramps and discomfort.
- **Supports Skin Health**: Chamomile tea's anti-inflammatory properties can also benefit the skin when applied topically, soothing irritated skin, eczema, and rashes.
- **Boosts Immune Function**: Drinking chamomile tea regularly may help boost the immune system, reducing the likelihood of catching colds or infections due to its mild antimicrobial properties.

Precautions:

Chamomile is generally considered safe for most people when consumed in moderate amounts. However, individuals with allergies to plants in the *Asteraceae* family (such as ragweed, daisies, or marigolds) should avoid chamomile, as it may trigger allergic reactions. Pregnant or breastfeeding women should consult a healthcare provider before using chamomile regularly, as it can stimulate uterine contractions in large amounts.

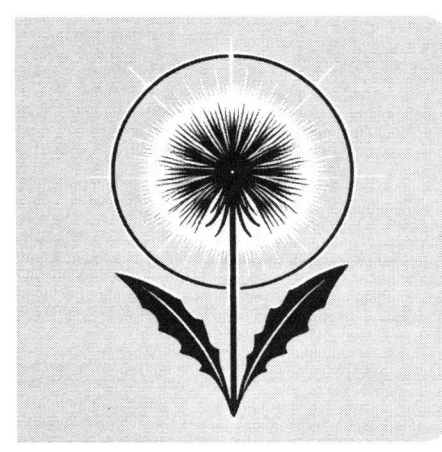

5. Dandelion Detox Salad

Dandelion Detox Salad is a nutritious and cleansing dish made from the leaves of the dandelion plant (*Taraxacum officinale*), which has long been revered for its detoxifying and health-boosting properties. Dandelion greens are packed with vitamins, minerals, and antioxidants, making them an excellent choice for supporting liver health, aiding digestion, and promoting overall wellness. This detox salad combines dandelion greens with other nutrient-dense ingredients to create a refreshing and flavorful meal that helps cleanse the body naturally.

Key Benefits of Dandelion Detox Salad:

- **Supports Liver Health**: Dandelion greens are known for their ability to promote liver detoxification. The bitter compounds in dandelion, such as *taraxacin*, stimulate bile production in the liver, which aids in the digestion and elimination of toxins from the body.
- **Diuretic Properties**: Dandelion acts as a natural diuretic, helping the body flush out excess water and toxins through increased urine production. This reduces bloating and supports kidney function.
- **Rich in Nutrients**: Dandelion greens are high in vitamins A, C, and K, as well as minerals like calcium, iron, and potassium. These nutrients support immune function, bone health, and overall vitality.
- **Antioxidant-Rich**: Dandelion contains powerful antioxidants, such as beta-carotene and polyphenols, which help neutralize free radicals, reduce inflammation, and protect cells from oxidative stress.
- **Aids Digestion**: The bitter taste of dandelion greens stimulates digestive enzymes and bile flow, improving digestion and reducing symptoms of indigestion and bloating.

Ingredients:
- 1 bunch fresh dandelion greens, washed and chopped (younger, tender greens are less bitter)
- 1 cup mixed greens (such as spinach, arugula, or kale)
- 1 avocado, sliced (for healthy fats)
- 1 small cucumber, sliced
- 1 radish, thinly sliced (for a peppery crunch)
- ¼ cup red onion, thinly sliced
- 2 tablespoons sunflower seeds or pumpkin seeds (for crunch and added nutrition)
- 1 tablespoon fresh lemon juice (for extra detox support)
- 2 tablespoons olive oil (for healthy fats)
- 1 teaspoon apple cider vinegar
- Salt and pepper to taste

How to Make a Dandelion Detox Salad:

Instructions:

1. Wash the dandelion greens thoroughly and chop them into bite-sized pieces. If you find the greens too bitter, you can blanch them briefly in boiling water for about 1-2 minutes, then rinse with cold water to reduce bitterness.
2. In a large salad bowl, combine the dandelion greens with mixed greens, cucumber, avocado, radish, and red onion.
3. In a small bowl, whisk together the olive oil, lemon juice, apple cider vinegar, salt, and pepper to make a light vinaigrette dressing.
4. Drizzle the dressing over the salad and toss to combine.
5. Sprinkle the sunflower seeds or pumpkin seeds on top for added texture and nutrients.
6. Serve immediately and enjoy the fresh, detoxifying flavors.

Nutritional and Detox Benefits of Key Ingredients:

- **Dandelion Greens**: These nutrient-dense leaves are a powerful detoxifier for the liver and kidneys. They contain high levels of vitamins A and C, which support skin health and boost immunity, while their diuretic properties help the body eliminate toxins naturally.
- **Avocado**: Rich in healthy monounsaturated fats and fiber, avocado supports digestion and aids the absorption of fat-soluble vitamins from the greens. Its creamy texture balances the bitterness of the dandelion.
- **Cucumber**: Cucumbers are hydrating and contain antioxidants like vitamin C and beta-carotene. Their high water content supports kidney function and helps flush out toxins.
- **Radish**: Radishes are another detoxifying vegetable, known for stimulating bile production and aiding digestion. They add a crunchy texture and peppery flavor to the salad.
- **Sunflower or Pumpkin Seeds**: These seeds are a great source of healthy fats, protein, and minerals like zinc and magnesium, which support immune function and reduce inflammation.

Health Benefits of Dandelion for Detoxification:

Liver Detoxification: Dandelion is highly regarded for its liver-cleansing properties. The bitter compounds in dandelion greens stimulate bile production, which is essential for breaking down fats and aiding in the elimination of toxins from the liver. This makes dandelion a valuable herb for promoting healthy liver function and preventing liver-related conditions like fatty liver disease.

Diuretic Action: Dandelion's diuretic properties help reduce water retention and eliminate excess waste through increased urination. Unlike synthetic diuretics, which can lead to a loss of important minerals, dandelion is naturally rich in potassium, which helps maintain a healthy electrolyte balance while promoting detoxification.

Rich in Antioxidants: Dandelion greens are abundant in antioxidants such as beta-carotene and polyphenols, which protect the body from oxidative stress and inflammation. These antioxidants help combat free radicals, which can cause cellular damage and contribute to chronic disease.

Variations and Additions:

- **Dandelion and Beet Salad**: Add roasted or grated beets to the salad for additional liver-supporting benefits. Beets contain betalains, which help detoxify the liver and improve bile flow.
- **Herb-Infused Dressing**: Incorporate detoxifying herbs like parsley or cilantro into the salad dressing to further support liver and kidney function.
- **Hard-Boiled Eggs**: Add hard-boiled eggs for a boost of protein and healthy fats, making the salad more filling and nutrient-rich.

Additional Benefits of Dandelion Detox Salad:

- **Supports Weight Loss**: The high fiber content in dandelion greens helps promote satiety, while the diuretic properties help reduce water retention, making this salad a great choice for those looking to support healthy weight management.
- **Promotes Skin Health**: The antioxidants and vitamin C in dandelion greens support collagen production and protect the skin from oxidative damage, promoting a healthy complexion.
- **Boosts Immune Function**: With its high levels of vitamins A and C, this salad strengthens the immune system by promoting the production of white blood cells and supporting overall immunity.

Precautions:

Dandelion greens are generally safe to eat, but individuals with allergies to plants in the *Asteraceae* family (such as ragweed, daisies, or marigolds) should exercise caution. Those with gallbladder problems or taking diuretic medications should consult with a healthcare provider before consuming large amounts of dandelion, as it may increase bile production or have diuretic effects.

chapter 4

Relieving Stress and Anxiety

- The Impact of Stress on Overall Health
- Top 5 Herbal Recipes for Calm and Relaxation
  1. Lavender Relaxation Tea
  2. Ashwagandha Stress Relief Tonic
  3. Valerian Root Sleep Aid
  4. Passionflower Calming Infusion
  5. Lemon Balm Serenity Syrup

The Impact of Stress on Overall Health

Stress has a profound impact on overall health, affecting both the body and mind in numerous ways. While stress is a natural response to challenging situations, chronic or unmanaged stress can lead to significant health problems over time. Stress triggers the body's "fight-or-flight" response, releasing hormones like cortisol and adrenaline that prepare the body to deal with immediate threats. However, when this response is activated frequently or for long periods, it can disrupt nearly every system in the body, leading to a range of physical and mental health issues.

Physical Impact of Stress:

1. **Cardiovascular System**: Chronic stress increases the risk of heart disease and hypertension. Stress causes an increase in heart rate and blood pressure as the body prepares for action. Over time, consistently elevated blood pressure can damage blood vessels and increase the risk of heart attack or stroke. Elevated stress hormones, particularly cortisol, also contribute to high cholesterol levels and the buildup of plaque in arteries.

2. **Immune System**: Stress weakens the immune system, making the body more susceptible to infections and diseases. Chronic stress suppresses the immune response by reducing the production of lymphocytes (white blood cells), which are essential for fighting infections. As a result, individuals under long-term stress are more likely to get sick frequently and may have a slower recovery time from illnesses.

3. **Digestive System**: Stress affects digestion in various ways, often exacerbating conditions like indigestion, acid reflux, irritable bowel syndrome (IBS), and gastritis. Stress hormones can alter the production of digestive enzymes and acids, slowing digestion or causing an overproduction of stomach acid, leading to heartburn or stomach ulcers. Chronic stress is also linked to changes in appetite, either increasing or decreasing it, which can contribute to weight fluctuations.

4. **Musculoskeletal System**: Stress causes muscle tension, particularly in the shoulders, neck, and back, leading to chronic pain or tension headaches. Prolonged muscle tension can also contribute to conditions such as tension-type headaches, migraines, or musculoskeletal disorders like fibromyalgia.

5. **Endocrine System**: Prolonged stress affects the endocrine system, which regulates hormones throughout the body. The continuous release of cortisol can lead to hormonal imbalances, contributing to weight gain, particularly around the abdomen, and increasing the risk of conditions like Type 2 diabetes due to insulin resistance.

6. **Reproductive Health**: In women, stress can disrupt menstrual cycles, causing irregular periods or exacerbating symptoms of premenstrual syndrome (PMS). High cortisol levels can interfere with the production of estrogen and progesterone, which can affect fertility. In men, stress can lower testosterone levels, reduce sperm production, and contribute to erectile dysfunction.

7. **Sleep Disorders**: Stress is a leading cause of sleep disorders, such as insomnia. Chronic stress disrupts the body's ability to fall asleep or stay asleep, often causing restless nights

Ch. 4 - Relieving Stress and Anxiety

or shallow sleep. Poor sleep exacerbates stress and creates a cycle of fatigue and anxiety, further impairing overall health.

Mental and Emotional Impact of Stress:

1. **Anxiety and Depression**: Stress is closely linked to mental health conditions such as anxiety and depression. Chronic stress can overwhelm the brain's ability to regulate mood and emotions, leading to persistent feelings of worry, fear, or sadness. Prolonged exposure to high levels of cortisol can also impair cognitive function, affecting memory and concentration, and contributing to feelings of hopelessness.

2. **Cognitive Impairment**: Stress impairs cognitive function by affecting areas of the brain like the hippocampus and prefrontal cortex, which are responsible for memory, learning, and decision-making. This can lead to difficulty concentrating, memory lapses, and reduced productivity.

3. **Emotional Dysregulation**: Stress often causes emotional dysregulation, making it difficult to manage emotions effectively. People under stress may experience mood swings, irritability, frustration, or anger. Over time, this can strain relationships and lead to social withdrawal.

4. **Burnout**: Chronic stress, particularly in work environments, can lead to burnout, a state of emotional, physical, and mental exhaustion caused by excessive and prolonged stress. Burnout is characterized by feelings of cynicism, detachment, and a sense of ineffectiveness, often resulting in reduced performance at work or in personal life.

Behavioral Impact of Stress:

1. **Unhealthy Coping Mechanisms**: Stress often leads people to adopt unhealthy coping mechanisms, such as overeating, smoking, alcohol consumption, or drug use. These behaviors may provide temporary relief but ultimately exacerbate health problems in the long term, contributing to obesity, addiction, or chronic diseases.

2. **Social Withdrawal**: Stress can affect interpersonal relationships by causing people to withdraw socially, avoiding friends and family, or becoming irritable and impatient with others. Over time, this isolation can lead to feelings of loneliness and contribute to the development of depression.

3. **Reduced Physical Activity**: Chronic stress often leads to fatigue and lack of motivation, which can reduce physical activity. This sedentary behavior further exacerbates health problems, such as weight gain, cardiovascular issues, and mood disorders.

Long-Term Health Consequences of Chronic Stress:

Chronic, unmanaged stress can lead to long-term health issues, including:

- **Heart Disease**: Prolonged stress is a significant risk factor for heart disease, increasing the likelihood of heart attacks and strokes due to constant high blood pressure and elevated cortisol levels.

- **Metabolic Disorders**: Stress is closely linked to metabolic conditions like obesity and Type 2 diabetes. Cortisol promotes the storage of fat, particularly around the abdomen, which increases the risk of developing insulin resistance.

- **Chronic Pain**: Stress-related muscle tension can lead to chronic pain conditions, including tension headaches, migraines, and musculoskeletal disorders.

- **Mental Health Disorders**: Anxiety, depression, and other mood disorders can develop or worsen under chronic stress, affecting overall quality of life.

Managing Stress for Better Health:

- **Mindfulness and Relaxation Techniques**: Practices like meditation, yoga, and deep breathing exercises can reduce the body's stress response, lowering cortisol levels and promoting relaxation.

- **Physical Activity**: Regular exercise helps manage stress by releasing endorphins, which improve mood and reduce anxiety. It also promotes better sleep and overall physical health.

- **Healthy Diet**: A balanced diet supports the body's ability to cope with stress by providing essential nutrients for brain and body function. Avoiding excessive sugar, caffeine, and alcohol can help stabilize mood and energy levels.

- **Social Support**: Maintaining strong relationships with family, friends, or support groups can provide emotional support during stressful times and reduce feelings of isolation.

Top 5 Herbal Recipes for Calm and Relaxation

Ch. 4 - Top 5 Herbal Recipes for Calm and Relaxation

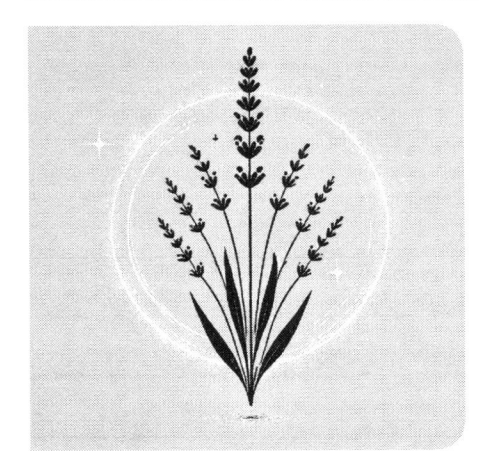

1. Lavender Relaxation Tea

Lavender Relaxation Tea is a soothing herbal infusion made from the dried flowers of the *Lavandula angustifolia* plant. Lavender has long been celebrated for its calming properties, making it an ideal remedy for reducing stress, promoting relaxation, and improving sleep quality. With its gentle floral aroma and mild taste, lavender tea can help relax the mind and body, ease tension, and support emotional well-being. This tea is perfect for those looking for a natural way to unwind, relieve anxiety, and prepare for restful sleep.

Key Benefits of Lavender Relaxation Tea:

- **Promotes Relaxation and Reduces Anxiety**: Lavender is well-known for its calming effects on the nervous system. It helps reduce symptoms of anxiety, tension, and stress by influencing neurotransmitters in the brain, particularly GABA, which promotes relaxation and reduces feelings of worry or nervousness.

- **Improves Sleep Quality**: Drinking lavender tea before bed can help calm the mind and prepare the body for a restful night's sleep. Lavender has mild sedative properties, making it useful for individuals suffering from insomnia or restlessness.

- **Relieves Headaches and Migraines**: Lavender's anti-inflammatory and calming properties make it effective for reducing headaches or migraines, especially those triggered by stress or tension.

- **Eases Digestive Discomfort**: Lavender has mild antispasmodic properties that help relax the muscles of the digestive tract, making it helpful for easing bloating, indigestion, or nausea, particularly when related to stress.

- **Supports Emotional Well-being**: The aromatic nature of lavender has a direct effect on the limbic system, the part of the brain that regulates emotions. This makes lavender tea a wonderful option for balancing mood and supporting emotional health.

How to Make Lavender Relaxation Tea:

Ingredients:
- 1 tablespoon dried lavender buds (or 1 teaspoon if using a stronger blend)
- 1 cup boiling water
- Optional: honey or lemon (for added sweetness or flavor)

Instructions:

1. Boil water and let it cool slightly (about 2-3 minutes after boiling).

2. Place the dried lavender buds in a tea strainer or directly into a teapot or mug.

3. Pour the hot water over the lavender buds and let the tea steep for 5-10 minutes, depending on how strong you prefer it.

4. Strain the tea or remove the strainer, and add honey or lemon if desired.

5. Sip the tea slowly, preferably in the evening or before bed, to help promote relaxation and calm.

Dosage:

- **For relaxation and anxiety relief**: Drink 1-2 cups of lavender tea daily, especially during periods of stress or in the evening to prepare for sleep.

- **For sleep support**: Drink 1 cup of lavender tea about 30 minutes before bedtime to calm the mind and promote restful sleep.

Science Behind Lavender's Relaxation Benefits:

Lavender's calming effects are attributed to its active compounds, particularly **linalool** and **linalyl acetate**, which have been shown to influence the central nervous system by reducing excitability and enhancing relaxation. Research indicates that these compounds increase the activity of the neurotransmitter **GABA**, which helps calm the nervous system and promotes relaxation, much like certain anti-anxiety medications. A study published in *Phytomedicine* found that lavender significantly reduced symptoms of generalized anxiety disorder, highlighting its effectiveness as a natural remedy for stress and anxiety.

Additionally, lavender has mild **sedative effects**, making it useful for those struggling with insomnia or restlessness. A study published in the *Journal of Alternative and Complementary Medicine* showed that inhaling lavender essential oil improved sleep quality in participants, while drinking lavender tea offers similar calming benefits.

Lavender's **anti-inflammatory** properties help reduce tension headaches and muscle soreness, especially when related to stress. By reducing inflammation and calming the nervous system, lavender promotes overall relaxation and well-being.

Variations and Additions:

- **Lavender and Chamomile Tea**: Combine lavender with chamomile flowers for an even stronger relaxation blend. Chamomile is well-known for its calming and sleep-inducing effects, making this combination ideal for evening use.
- **Lavender and Peppermint Tea**: Add fresh peppermint leaves for a refreshing, cooling tea that supports digestion and soothes tension headaches while also promoting relaxation.
- **Lavender and Lemon Balm Tea**: Lemon balm is another calming herb that works well with lavender. It helps reduce stress and anxiety, making the tea a powerful mood-balancing blend.
- **Lavender and Ginger Tea**: For an added anti-inflammatory boost and digestive support, add fresh ginger slices to your lavender tea. Ginger's warming properties complement lavender's relaxing effects, especially after meals.

Additional Benefits of Lavender Relaxation Tea:

- **Supports Respiratory Health**: Lavender's anti-inflammatory and antimicrobial properties can help soothe respiratory issues like a sore throat or mild cough, particularly when caused by irritation or stress.
- **Boosts Skin Health**: Drinking lavender tea can have indirect benefits for the skin by reducing inflammation and stress, which are common triggers for conditions like acne, eczema, or psoriasis.
- **Reduces Menstrual Pain**: Lavender's antispasmodic properties can help ease menstrual cramps by relaxing the muscles of the uterus. Drinking lavender tea during menstruation may provide relief from discomfort and tension.

Precautions:

While lavender tea is generally safe for most people, individuals with allergies to lavender or plants in the *Lamiaceae* family (such as mint or sage) should avoid using it. Pregnant and breastfeeding women should consult with a healthcare provider before consuming lavender regularly, as it may affect hormone levels or cause uterine stimulation in high doses.

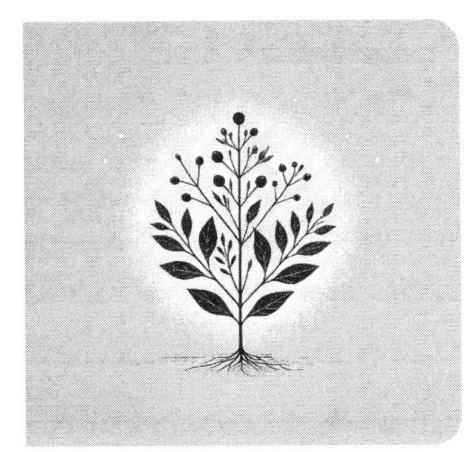

2. Ashwagandha Stress Relief Tonic

Ashwagandha Stress Relief Tonic is a powerful herbal remedy that uses *Withania somnifera*, commonly known as ashwagandha, to help reduce stress, balance cortisol levels, and promote overall well-being. Ashwagandha is an adaptogen, meaning it helps the body cope with physical, emotional, and environmental stress by supporting the adrenal glands and regulating the body's stress response. It has been used for centuries in Ayurvedic medicine for its rejuvenating and calming properties, making it an ideal choice for reducing chronic stress, enhancing mental clarity, and supporting physical resilience.

Key Benefits of Ashwagandha Stress Relief Tonic:

- **Reduces Stress and Anxiety**: Ashwagandha helps lower cortisol, the stress hormone, which is often elevated during periods of chronic stress. This tonic helps the body adapt to stressful situations, promoting a sense of calm and reducing symptoms of anxiety.
- **Balances Cortisol Levels**: Chronic stress can lead to consistently high cortisol levels, which can negatively affect sleep, energy levels, and overall health. Ashwagandha has been shown to help regulate cortisol, preventing the harmful effects of prolonged stress.
- **Promotes Mental Clarity and Focus**: By reducing stress and calming the nervous system, ashwagandha improves focus, concentration, and cognitive function, helping to clear mental fog and increase productivity.
- **Supports Adrenal Function**: As an adaptogen, ashwagandha helps support and protect the adrenal glands, preventing adrenal fatigue caused by prolonged exposure to stress. It helps restore balance to the body's stress-response system.
- **Enhances Sleep Quality**: Ashwagandha's calming effects make it useful for improving sleep quality. It helps relax the mind and body, making it easier to fall asleep and stay asleep, especially for those dealing with insomnia or restlessness.

How to Make Ashwagandha Stress Relief Tonic:

Ingredients:
- 1 teaspoon ashwagandha powder (organic and pure)
- 1 cup warm almond milk (or another plant-based milk)
- ½ teaspoon honey or maple syrup (optional, for sweetness)
- ¼ teaspoon cinnamon (optional, for flavor and anti-inflammatory benefits)
- ¼ teaspoon ground turmeric (optional, for additional calming and anti-inflammatory properties)

Instructions:

1. Warm the almond milk in a small saucepan over low heat. Be careful not to let it boil, as you want the milk to stay warm but not too hot.
2. Add the ashwagandha powder, cinnamon, and turmeric (if using), and whisk until fully dissolved and combined.
3. Remove from heat and stir in the honey or maple syrup to add sweetness, if desired.
4. Pour the tonic into a cup and sip slowly, preferably in the evening or during moments of stress for its calming effects.

Dosage:

- **For stress relief**: Drink 1 cup of ashwagandha tonic daily, particularly in the evening, to help lower stress and support relaxation.
- **For adrenal support**: Consume 1 cup daily over an extended period (4-6 weeks) to help balance cortisol levels and support adrenal health.

Science Behind Ashwagandha's Stress-Relieving Benefits:

Ashwagandha has been extensively studied for its ability to reduce stress and anxiety. One of its primary active compounds, **withanolides**, has adaptogenic properties that help modulate the body's stress response by balancing cortisol levels. A study published in the *Indian Journal of Psychological Medicine* found that participants who took ashwagandha supplements experienced a significant reduction in cortisol levels and perceived stress compared to those in the placebo group.

Additionally, ashwagandha is known to support the **hypothalamic-pituitary-adrenal (HPA) axis**, which is responsible for regulating the body's response to stress. By supporting this system, ashwagandha helps prevent the adrenal glands from becoming overworked, a condition known as **adrenal fatigue**, which is common in individuals experiencing prolonged stress.

Ashwagandha has also been shown to improve **cognitive function**, reduce symptoms of **anxiety** and **depression**, and promote a general sense of well-being. Its ability to calm the nervous system makes it particularly effective for those suffering from chronic stress or stress-related disorders.

Variations and Additions:

- **Ashwagandha and Ginger Tonic**: Add fresh ginger slices or a small amount of ground ginger to your tonic for its anti-inflammatory properties and digestive benefits. Ginger also enhances circulation and warmth, making this version ideal for cold or stress-induced fatigue.
- **Ashwagandha and Chamomile Tonic**: Combine ashwagandha with chamomile for an even more calming effect. Chamomile is known for its sedative properties and helps promote better sleep, making this combination great for evening relaxation.
- **Ashwagandha Golden Milk**: Add a full teaspoon of turmeric and a pinch of black pepper to create a golden milk version of the tonic. Turmeric has powerful anti-inflammatory properties, and black pepper enhances the absorption of turmeric's active compound, curcumin.

Additional Benefits of Ashwagandha:

- **Boosts Immune Function**: Ashwagandha has immunomodulatory effects, helping to strengthen the immune system and protect the body from illness. It also reduces inflammation, which supports overall immune health.
- **Enhances Physical Stamina**: Ashwagandha is commonly used to enhance endurance and physical stamina, making it a popular herb for athletes or those recovering from physical exhaustion. It helps improve energy levels and reduce fatigue.
- **Balances Hormones**: Ashwagandha supports hormonal balance, particularly by regulating cortisol and thyroid function. This makes it helpful for those with thyroid imbalances, such as hypothyroidism.
- **Supports Heart Health**: Some studies suggest that ashwagandha may help lower cholesterol and blood pressure, contributing to better cardiovascular health.

Precautions:

pregnant women should avoid using ashwagandha, as it may cause uterine contractions. Individuals with autoimmune conditions, such as lupus or rheumatoid arthritis, should consult with a healthcare provider before using ashwagandha, as it may stimulate the immune system. People taking medications for thyroid disorders or blood pressure should also seek advice from a healthcare professional, as ashwagandha can interact with these medications.

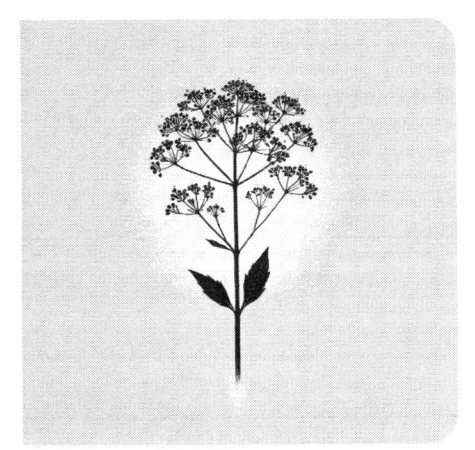

3. Valerian Root Sleep Aid

Valerian Root Sleep Aid is a natural herbal remedy made from the root of the *Valeriana officinalis* plant, which has been used for centuries to promote relaxation and improve sleep quality. Valerian root is particularly well-known for its calming effects on the nervous system, making it an effective remedy for insomnia, anxiety, and restlessness. Unlike some sleep medications, valerian root works gently to help you fall asleep naturally without causing grogginess or dependency.

Key Benefits of Valerian Root Sleep Aid:

- **Promotes Restful Sleep**: Valerian root is one of the most popular herbs for treating insomnia and improving overall sleep quality. It helps reduce the time it takes to fall asleep and improves the depth of sleep, allowing for a more restful night.
- **Reduces Anxiety and Stress**: Valerian has calming properties that help reduce symptoms of anxiety, restlessness, and stress, which are common contributors to sleep disturbances. By calming the mind and body, it helps you unwind and relax before bedtime.
- **Improves Sleep Without Grogginess**: Unlike many synthetic sleep aids, valerian root does not leave you feeling groggy or drowsy the next morning. Its effects are mild, allowing for a more natural sleep cycle.
- **Eases Muscle Tension and Cramps**: Valerian root has mild muscle-relaxing properties, which can be helpful for those who experience muscle tension or cramps that interfere with sleep.
- **Non-Habit Forming**: Valerian root is a natural remedy and is generally considered non-habit-forming, making it a safer alternative to many pharmaceutical sleep medications.

How to Make Valerian Root Sleep Aid Tea:

Ingredients:
- 1 teaspoon dried valerian root (or 1 valerian tea bag)
- 1 cup boiling water
- Optional: honey or chamomile (for added sweetness and calming benefits)

Instructions:

1. Boil water and let it cool slightly for 2-3 minutes before pouring it over the valerian root.
2. Place the valerian root or tea bag in a teapot or mug.
3. Pour the hot water over the valerian root and cover the mug to retain the aromatic compounds.
4. Let the tea steep for 10-15 minutes to allow the valerian root to fully release its beneficial properties.
5. Strain the tea if using loose valerian root and add honey or chamomile if desired for flavor.
6. Drink the tea about 30 minutes to an hour before bedtime for best results.

Dosage:

- **For sleep support**: Drink 1 cup of valerian root tea 30-60 minutes before bed to help induce sleep and improve sleep quality.

- **For anxiety and relaxation**: Drink 1 cup as needed during periods of high stress or anxiety to promote calmness and reduce tension.

Science Behind Valerian Root's Sleep Benefits:

Valerian root contains several compounds, including **valerenic acid**, **isovaleric acid**, and **valepotriates**, which work together to promote relaxation and sleep. These compounds are believed to interact with **GABA (gamma-aminobutyric acid)** receptors in the brain. GABA is a neurotransmitter that reduces nervous system activity, helping to calm the mind and body. By increasing GABA levels, valerian root helps reduce anxiety, stress, and hyperactivity, leading to better sleep.

Several studies support the use of valerian root for improving sleep quality. A study published in *Phytomedicine* found that valerian root significantly improved sleep latency (the time it takes to fall asleep) and sleep quality without causing morning grogginess. Another study in *BMC Complementary Medicine and Therapies* confirmed that valerian root improved sleep quality in individuals suffering from mild insomnia, particularly when taken over several weeks.

Variations and Additions:

- **Valerian and Chamomile Tea**: Add 1 teaspoon of dried chamomile flowers to your valerian tea for a soothing combination. Chamomile enhances the calming effects of valerian, making this blend perfect for winding down at the end of the day.
- **Valerian and Lavender Tea**: For extra relaxation, combine valerian with lavender flowers. Lavender is known for its ability to promote calm and improve sleep quality, adding a pleasant aroma and flavor to the tea.
- **Valerian and Lemon Balm Tea**: Lemon balm is another herb commonly used for reducing anxiety and promoting restful sleep. Mixing it with valerian root creates a more potent sleep aid that also helps ease digestive discomforts that might interfere with sleep.
- **Valerian Root Tincture**: If you prefer a more concentrated form of valerian, you can use a valerian root tincture. Add 1-2 droppers of the tincture to a glass of water or tea before bed for similar effects.

Additional Benefits of Valerian Root:

- **Helps with Anxiety**: Valerian root is not only a sleep aid but also an effective remedy for anxiety. Its ability to increase GABA levels makes it useful for those who experience anxiety during the day, helping to ease tension and promote calm without sedation.
- **Eases PMS Symptoms**: Valerian's antispasmodic and muscle-relaxing properties make it helpful for relieving menstrual cramps and other symptoms of premenstrual syndrome (PMS). Drinking valerian tea during the menstrual cycle may help reduce discomfort.
- **Supports Nervous System Health**: Regular use of valerian root can help calm the nervous system, reducing the long-term effects of chronic stress, such as fatigue, muscle tension, and irritability.

Precautions:

While valerian root is generally safe for most people when used in moderation, there are a few precautions to keep in mind:

- **Pregnancy and breastfeeding**: Pregnant or breastfeeding women should avoid valerian root, as its safety during pregnancy has not been well-studied.
- **Long-term use**: While valerian is non-habit forming, it's best to use it for short periods (up to a few weeks) and consult with a healthcare provider if needed for longer use.
- **Sedative effects**: Valerian root can have sedative effects, so it's important not to combine it with alcohol, sedative medications, or other substances that induce drowsiness, as this may amplify the effects.
- **Grogginess**: Though uncommon, some individuals may experience mild grogginess or a "hangover" effect the next morning after using valerian. If this occurs, try reducing the dosage or discontinuing use.

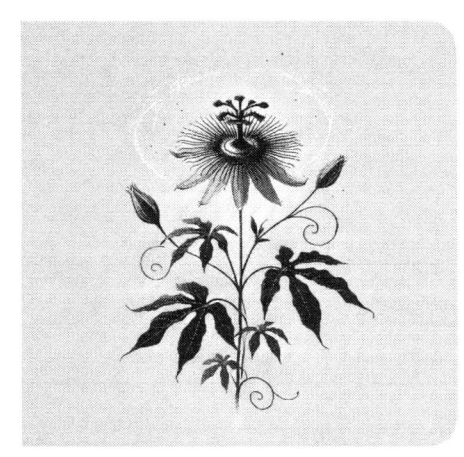

4. Passionflower Calming Infusion

Passionflower Calming Infusion is a soothing herbal tea made from the dried flowers, stems, and leaves of the *Passiflora incarnata* plant. Known for its calming effects, passionflower has been used for centuries to ease anxiety, promote relaxation, and improve sleep quality. It works by increasing levels of gamma-aminobutyric acid (GABA) in the brain, a neurotransmitter that helps calm the nervous system and reduce stress. This calming infusion is ideal for those dealing with anxiety, stress, or insomnia, offering a natural, non-habit-forming way to unwind and find balance.

Key Benefits of Passionflower Calming Infusion:

- **Reduces Anxiety and Stress**: Passionflower is widely used to help manage anxiety and reduce stress. By increasing GABA levels in the brain, passionflower helps lower nervous system activity, providing a natural way to calm racing thoughts and ease tension.
- **Promotes Restful Sleep**: Passionflower is particularly effective for improving sleep quality, especially for those who experience insomnia or restlessness due to anxiety. It helps shorten the time it takes to fall asleep and improves the depth and duration of sleep without causing grogginess the next morning.
- **Eases Muscle Tension**: Passionflower has mild antispasmodic properties, which help relax muscles and relieve tension. This makes it helpful for reducing stress-related muscle aches and cramping, allowing for a deeper state of relaxation.
- **Balances Mood**: Passionflower's calming effect on the nervous system helps stabilize mood, making it beneficial for those experiencing mood swings, irritability, or emotional imbalances related to stress or anxiety.
- **Supports Mental Clarity**: While passionflower is calming, it does not impair cognitive function. In fact, by reducing anxiety and tension, it may help improve focus and mental clarity, especially for those whose anxiety interferes with concentration.

How to Make Passionflower Calming Infusion:

Ingredients:
- 1 teaspoon dried passionflower (or 1 passionflower tea bag)
- 1 cup boiling water
- Optional: honey or lemon (for added flavor and benefits)

Instructions:

1. Bring water to a boil and let it cool slightly for 2-3 minutes.
2. Place the dried passionflower in a tea infuser or directly in a mug.
3. Pour the hot water over the passionflower, covering it completely.
4. Allow the tea to steep for 10-15 minutes, depending on your desired strength.
5. Strain the tea or remove the tea bag, and add honey or lemon if desired.
6. Sip slowly, preferably in the evening or whenever you need to relax.

Dosage:

- **For anxiety and relaxation**: Drink 1-2 cups of passionflower tea daily, especially during stressful times or in the evening to promote relaxation.

- **For sleep support**: Drink 1 cup of passionflower tea 30-60 minutes before bed to help improve sleep quality and reduce restlessness.

Science Behind Fennel's Digestive Benefits:

Passionflower's ability to reduce anxiety and promote relaxation is primarily due to its effect on **GABA** levels in the brain. **GABA (gamma-aminobutyric acid)** is a neurotransmitter that inhibits overactivity in the brain, calming the nervous system and reducing feelings of stress and anxiety. Passionflower increases GABA availability, helping to induce a sense of calm and well-being. Research has shown that passionflower can be as effective as certain anxiety medications in reducing symptoms of generalized anxiety disorder, but without the risk of dependency.

A study published in the *Journal of Clinical Pharmacy and Therapeutics* found that passionflower was effective in reducing anxiety in patients undergoing surgery, demonstrating its strong calming properties. Another study in *Phytotherapy Research* showed that passionflower significantly improved sleep quality in individuals suffering from mild insomnia.

Variations and Additions:

- **Passionflower and Chamomile Tea**: Blend passionflower with chamomile for an extra calming effect. Chamomile also has sedative and anti-anxiety properties, making this combination ideal for those seeking deep relaxation and sleep support.
- **Passionflower and Lemon Balm Tea**: Add lemon balm to your passionflower tea to enhance its calming effects. Lemon balm is known for reducing anxiety and improving mood, complementing passionflower's relaxing qualities.
- **Passionflower and Lavender Tea**: Combine passionflower with lavender flowers for a floral, soothing blend that enhances both relaxation and sleep. Lavender's aromatic compounds are known to reduce stress and promote tranquility.
- **Passionflower and Peppermint Tea**: For a refreshing twist, add peppermint leaves to your passionflower infusion. Peppermint helps relieve tension headaches and aids digestion, making it a perfect addition to this calming tea.

Additional Benefits of Passionflower:

- **Supports Heart Health**: Some studies suggest that passionflower may help lower blood pressure by reducing stress and relaxing the blood vessels. Its calming effect on the nervous system can contribute to better cardiovascular health over time.
- **Eases PMS Symptoms**: Passionflower's ability to reduce tension and ease mood swings makes it helpful for women dealing with premenstrual syndrome (PMS). It can also reduce cramps and irritability related to hormonal fluctuations.
- **Soothes Digestive Discomfort**: Passionflower's antispasmodic properties can help relax the digestive tract, making it useful for those who experience stress-induced digestive issues like cramping, bloating, or indigestion.

Precautions:

While passionflower is generally safe for most people, it's important to take a few precautions:
- **Pregnancy and breastfeeding**: Pregnant or breastfeeding women should consult with a healthcare provider before using passionflower, as its effects during pregnancy are not well studied.
- **Sedative effects**: Passionflower has mild sedative properties, so it's important not to combine it with alcohol, sedatives, or other substances that cause drowsiness.
- **Medication interactions**: If you are taking medications for anxiety, depression, or insomnia, consult with a healthcare provider before using passionflower, as it may enhance the effects of these medications.

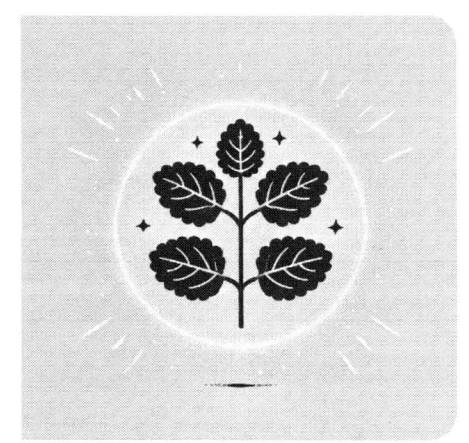

5. Lemon Balm Serenity Syrup

Lemon Balm Serenity Syrup is a soothing herbal remedy made from the leaves of the lemon balm plant (*Melissa officinalis*), a member of the mint family known for its calming and mood-enhancing properties. This syrup can be used to reduce anxiety, promote relaxation, and improve sleep quality, making it an excellent natural remedy for those experiencing stress, restlessness, or insomnia. With its pleasant, mild lemon flavor, lemon balm syrup is easy to incorporate into daily routines and can be enjoyed on its own or added to teas and beverages.

Key Benefits of Lemon Balm Serenity Syrup:

- **Reduces Anxiety and Stress**: Lemon balm has been traditionally used to ease anxiety and calm the nervous system. Its active compounds, such as **rosmarinic acid**, help balance neurotransmitters like GABA, which promotes relaxation and reduces feelings of nervousness.
- **Promotes Restful Sleep**: Lemon balm is particularly effective in improving sleep quality. By calming the mind and reducing stress, it helps prepare the body for sleep and can shorten the time it takes to fall asleep. It's especially useful for those experiencing insomnia due to stress or anxiety.
- **Improves Mood**: Lemon balm has mild antidepressant properties, helping to lift mood and ease symptoms of mild depression. Its calming effects also help stabilize emotional responses, making it beneficial for emotional balance.
- **Supports Digestive Health**: Lemon balm is known for its ability to soothe digestive discomfort, particularly when it is caused by stress. It helps relieve bloating, cramping, and indigestion, especially when taken before or after meals.
- **Gentle and Non-Habit Forming**: Lemon balm is a gentle herb that can be used regularly without causing dependency or drowsiness. Its calming effects are subtle, making it suitable for both daytime use to ease anxiety and evening use to promote sleep.

How to Make Lemon Balm Serenity Syrup:

Ingredients:
- 1 cup fresh lemon balm leaves (or ½ cup dried lemon balm)
- 2 cups water
- 1 cup raw honey (or maple syrup for a vegan option)
- Optional: 1 teaspoon fresh lemon juice (for extra flavor and calming benefits)

Instructions:

1. In a saucepan, bring the water to a boil, then reduce the heat to low.
2. Add the fresh or dried lemon balm leaves to the water and simmer for about 20 minutes, allowing the herbs to infuse fully.
3. Remove the saucepan from the heat and let the mixture cool slightly. Strain out the lemon balm leaves, pressing gently to extract all the liquid.
4. Stir in the honey or maple syrup until it dissolves completely in the warm liquid.
5. If desired, add the lemon juice for an extra calming and flavor boost.
6. Pour the syrup into a clean glass jar or bottle and store it in the refrigerator for up to 2 weeks.

Dosage:

- **For anxiety and stress relief**: Take 1-2 teaspoons of lemon balm syrup as needed throughout the day, especially during times of stress or nervousness.
- **For sleep support**: Take 1-2 teaspoons about 30 minutes before bedtime to help calm the mind and prepare for restful sleep.
- **For digestive health**: Take 1 teaspoon before or after meals to ease digestive discomfort related to stress.

Science Behind Lemon Balm's Calming Effects:

Lemon balm is rich in **rosmarinic acid**, a compound that increases the availability of **GABA (gamma-aminobutyric acid)**, a neurotransmitter that helps calm the nervous system. GABA reduces excitability in the brain, promoting a state of relaxation and reducing anxiety. Studies have shown that lemon balm can help ease symptoms of **generalized anxiety disorder** and **stress**, making it a valuable herb for emotional balance.

A study published in *Phytotherapy Research* found that individuals who consumed lemon balm experienced significant improvements in mood and cognitive function, with reduced feelings of anxiety. Lemon balm has also been shown to improve **sleep quality** in individuals suffering from insomnia, particularly when taken in the evening to help the body relax.

Variations and Additions:

- **Lemon Balm and Chamomile Syrup**: Combine lemon balm with chamomile flowers for an even more calming and sleep-promoting syrup. Chamomile enhances the sedative effects of lemon balm, making this variation ideal for nighttime use.
- **Lemon Balm and Lavender Syrup**: Add a few sprigs of lavender to the lemon balm infusion for a floral, aromatic twist. Lavender complements lemon balm's relaxing effects and adds a pleasant fragrance.
- **Lemon Balm and Ginger Syrup**: For a digestive and warming boost, add fresh ginger slices to the lemon balm infusion. Ginger enhances digestion and reduces nausea, particularly when stress affects the stomach.
- **Lemon Balm and Valerian Root Syrup**: If stronger relaxation or sleep support is needed, add a small amount of valerian root to the lemon balm infusion. Valerian is known for its sedative effects and can help with more severe cases of insomnia or anxiety.

Additional Benefits of Lemon Balm:

- **Boosts Cognitive Function**: Lemon balm has been shown to improve focus, memory, and cognitive performance. It helps reduce mental fatigue, making it useful for those who need to stay sharp during stressful situations.
- **Antiviral Properties**: Lemon balm has antiviral effects and may help protect against common viral infections, including cold sores caused by the herpes simplex virus.
- **Hormonal Balance**: Lemon balm can help ease symptoms of hormonal imbalances, particularly those associated with menopause and PMS, by reducing mood swings, irritability, and tension.

Precautions:

Lemon balm is generally safe for most people when consumed in moderate amounts. However, individuals with thyroid disorders, particularly hypothyroidism, should consult a healthcare provider before using lemon balm regularly, as it may affect thyroid hormone levels. Pregnant or breastfeeding women should also consult with a healthcare provider before using lemon balm in large amounts.

Chapter 5

Supporting Respiratory Health

- Understanding Respiratory Ailments
- Top 5 Herbal Recipes for Respiratory Support
  1. Eucalyptus Steam Inhalation
  2. Mullein Lung Tea
  3. Thyme Cough Syrup
  4. Licorice Root Respiratory Tonic
  5. Peppermint Chest Balm

Understanding Respiratory Ailments

Understanding Respiratory Ailments involves exploring the conditions that affect the respiratory system, including the lungs, airways, and associated structures. The respiratory system is essential for breathing, providing oxygen to the body and expelling carbon dioxide. When it is compromised by illness or external factors, a variety of respiratory ailments can arise, ranging from mild issues such as the common cold to more severe chronic diseases like asthma and chronic obstructive pulmonary disease (COPD).

Key Components of the Respiratory System:

1. **Nasal Passages and Sinuses**: These filter, warm, and humidify air as it enters the body.

2. **Pharynx and Larynx**: The throat and voice box help in swallowing and protecting the airway from food or liquids.

3. **Trachea and Bronchi**: The windpipe (trachea) and its branches (bronchi) transport air to the lungs.

4. **Lungs and Alveoli**: The lungs contain millions of tiny air sacs (alveoli) where gas exchange occurs – oxygen enters the blood, and carbon dioxide is removed.

When any part of this system is disrupted or infected, respiratory ailments occur.

Common Respiratory Ailments:

1. **Upper Respiratory Infections (URIs)**: These infections primarily affect the nose, throat, and sinuses, with the most common examples being the **common cold, sinusitis,** and **laryngitis**. Symptoms include a runny nose, sore throat, coughing, and sneezing. Viral infections are usually the cause, but bacterial infections can also occur.

2. **Lower Respiratory Infections (LRIs)**: These involve the lungs and airways, with conditions like **bronchitis** and **pneumonia** being common examples. LRIs can cause more severe symptoms, such as deep coughing, chest pain, and difficulty breathing.

3. **Asthma**: A chronic condition characterized by inflammation and narrowing of the airways. Asthma leads to symptoms such as wheezing, shortness of breath, chest tightness, and coughing. Triggers include allergens, exercise, cold air, and stress.

4. **Chronic Obstructive Pulmonary Disease (COPD)**: COPD is a progressive condition that includes **chronic bronchitis** and **emphysema**, where airflow is obstructed, leading to breathing difficulties. Symptoms include persistent cough, mucus production, and shortness of breath. Smoking is a leading cause of COPD.

5. **Allergic Rhinitis (Hay Fever)**: This occurs when the immune system overreacts to airborne allergens like pollen, dust mites, or pet dander, causing sneezing, congestion, and watery eyes.

6. **Influenza (Flu)**: A viral infection that affects the respiratory system more severely than a common cold. The flu can lead to high fever, body aches, fatigue, and in severe cases, pneumonia or hospitalization, especially in vulnerable populations.

7. **Pulmonary Fibrosis**: A condition characterized by scarring of the lung tissue, leading to stiffness and difficulty in breathing. It can be caused by environmental factors like long-term exposure to toxins, radiation, or as a side effect of certain medications.

8. **Tuberculosis (TB)**: Caused by the bacteria *Mycobacterium tuberculosis*, this disease primarily affects the lungs, leading to symptoms like a persistent cough, chest pain, and coughing up blood. TB spreads through the air and is a major global health concern.

9. **Lung Cancer**: This condition often results from smoking or exposure to harmful substances like asbestos or radon. Symptoms include persistent cough, weight loss, and chest pain. Early detection significantly improves the outcome.

Causes and Risk Factors for Respiratory Ailments:

- **Infections**: Viral, bacterial, and fungal infections can cause a range of respiratory issues, from mild colds to life-threatening pneumonia.

- **Smoking**: Cigarette smoke is a leading cause of chronic respiratory conditions such as COPD, emphysema, and lung cancer.

- **Pollutants and Toxins**: Long-term exposure to air pollution, industrial chemicals, and environmental toxins increases the risk of respiratory diseases.

- **Allergens**: Exposure to pollen, mold, dust mites, and pet dander can trigger allergic reactions and conditions like asthma or allergic rhinitis.

- **Genetics**: Family history plays a role in conditions like asthma, cystic fibrosis, and certain forms of pulmonary fibrosis.

- **Age and Immune Function**: Children, the elderly, and those with weakened immune systems are more susceptible to respiratory infections and complications.

Symptoms of Respiratory Ailments:

- **Coughing** (dry or productive with mucus)

- **Wheezing** (a whistling sound when breathing)

- **Shortness of breath** (dyspnea)

- **Chest pain or tightness**

- **Fatigue** and **weakness**

- **Fever** (in case of infections like flu or pneumonia)

- **Sore throat**
- **Nasal congestion** or **runny nose**

Diagnosis of Respiratory Conditions:

- **Physical Examination**: A healthcare provider will assess breathing patterns, check for wheezing or abnormal lung sounds, and evaluate overall health.
- **Chest X-rays or CT Scans**: These imaging tests can help detect conditions like pneumonia, TB, lung cancer, or fluid in the lungs.
- **Spirometry**: This test measures lung function, specifically how much air you can inhale and exhale, helping to diagnose conditions like asthma and COPD.
- **Blood Tests**: These can reveal infections, immune responses, or other health markers linked to respiratory conditions.
- **Sputum Tests**: Analyzing mucus can help identify infections, such as bacterial pneumonia or TB.

Treatment of Respiratory Ailments:

- **Medications**: Treatments include **antibiotics** for bacterial infections, **antiviral drugs** for viral infections like influenza, and **inhalers** or **bronchodilators** for conditions like asthma or COPD.
- **Corticosteroids**: These are often prescribed to reduce inflammation in conditions like asthma or severe allergic reactions.
- **Oxygen Therapy**: For chronic conditions like COPD, oxygen therapy may be needed to improve breathing and quality of life.
- **Pulmonary Rehabilitation**: A structured program of exercise, education, and support to help people with chronic lung diseases improve their physical condition and breathing.
- **Lifestyle Changes**: Quitting smoking, reducing exposure to allergens, and avoiding air pollutants are critical steps in preventing or managing respiratory diseases.
- **Vaccination**: Annual flu shots and pneumonia vaccines help protect vulnerable populations from severe respiratory infections.

Prevention of Respiratory Ailments:

- **Quit Smoking**: Avoiding or quitting smoking is the single most effective way to prevent respiratory diseases, including COPD and lung cancer.
- **Limit Exposure to Pollutants**: Minimize time spent in areas with high air pollution, use protective gear if working in environments with harmful chemicals, and ensure proper ventilation in homes and workplaces.
- **Vaccinations**: Stay up to date on vaccines, especially for the flu and pneumonia, to reduce the risk of severe respiratory infections.

Ch. 5 - Supporting Respiratory Health

- **Practice Good Hygiene**: Washing hands frequently, covering the mouth when coughing or sneezing, and avoiding close contact with sick individuals can help prevent the spread of infections.

- **Manage Allergies**: Controlling exposure to allergens like dust, pollen, and pet dander helps prevent allergic rhinitis and asthma flare-ups.

- **Healthy Diet and Exercise**: A balanced diet rich in antioxidants and regular physical activity can strengthen the immune system and improve lung function.

Top 5
Herbal Recipes for Respiratory Support

1. Eucalyptus Steam Inhalation

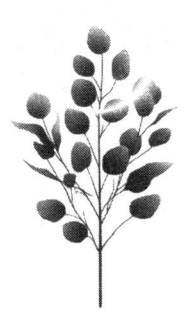

Eucalyptus Steam Inhalation is a natural and effective remedy used to relieve symptoms of respiratory ailments such as nasal congestion, sinusitis, and bronchitis. Eucalyptus oil, extracted from the leaves of the *Eucalyptus globulus* tree, contains a compound called **eucalyptol (cineole)**, which has anti-inflammatory, antiviral, antibacterial, and decongestant properties. When used in steam inhalation, eucalyptus oil helps open the airways, soothe irritated tissues, and clear mucus, providing relief from respiratory discomfort.

Key Benefits of Eucalyptus Steam Inhalation:

- **Clears Nasal Congestion**: Eucalyptus oil acts as a natural decongestant, helping to open blocked nasal passages. It thins mucus, making it easier to expel, which is especially beneficial during colds, sinus infections, and allergies.

- **Relieves Sinus Pressure**: The warm steam helps soothe inflamed sinuses, while eucalyptus oil's anti-inflammatory properties reduce swelling in the sinus cavities, providing relief from pressure and headaches.

- **Soothes Respiratory Inflammation**: Eucalyptus helps calm inflammation in the respiratory tract, making it useful for conditions like bronchitis and asthma. Its ability to reduce swelling and improve airflow can make breathing easier during respiratory flare-ups.

- **Antimicrobial Properties**: Eucalyptus oil has antiviral and antibacterial effects, which may help reduce the severity of colds and other respiratory infections by inhibiting the growth of harmful microbes.

- **Promotes Relaxation**: In addition to its respiratory benefits, the invigorating aroma of eucalyptus oil can also help reduce stress and promote relaxation, making steam inhalation a soothing ritual.

How to Perform Eucalyptus Steam Inhalation:

Ingredients:
- 4-5 drops of eucalyptus essential oil
- A large bowl of hot (but not boiling) water
- A towel

Instructions:

1. Boil water and let it cool slightly before pouring it into a large bowl. The water should be hot enough to produce steam but not so hot that it causes burns.

2. Add 4-5 drops of eucalyptus essential oil to the hot water.

3. Place a towel over your head to create a tent, then lean over the bowl, keeping your face at a safe distance from the water (about 10-12 inches).

4. Close your eyes and breathe in deeply through your nose, inhaling the eucalyptus-infused steam. Continue inhaling for 5-10 minutes, taking breaks if needed.

5. After the steam session, gently blow your nose to expel loosened mucus, and drink a glass of water to stay hydrated.

Dosage and Frequency:

- **For congestion relief**: Perform eucalyptus steam inhalation once or twice daily when experiencing nasal congestion, sinusitis, or bronchitis. For mild cases, once a day may suffice.

- **For chronic conditions**: Use the steam inhalation method as needed, especially during asthma flare-ups or allergies, but consult with a healthcare provider for long-term use.

Science Behind Eucalyptus Oil's Benefits:

Eucalyptus oil's main active compound, **eucalyptol (cineole)**, has been studied for its ability to reduce inflammation and mucus production in the airways. Research published in the *Journal of Ethnopharmacology* found that eucalyptol can improve symptoms of sinusitis by reducing nasal congestion and thinning mucus, making it easier to expel.

Additionally, eucalyptol has antimicrobial properties, which may help reduce the viral and bacterial load in respiratory infections. Studies have shown that eucalyptus oil can inhibit the growth of **bacteria** such as *Staphylococcus aureus* and **viruses** like the flu virus, supporting its use as a complementary treatment for colds and respiratory infections.

Variations and Additions:

- **Eucalyptus and Peppermint Steam**: Add 1-2 drops of peppermint essential oil to the eucalyptus steam for an extra cooling and decongestant effect. Peppermint oil contains menthol, which can enhance the soothing and respiratory-clearing benefits.

- **Eucalyptus and Lavender Steam**: For a calming and relaxing effect, add a few drops of lavender essential oil. Lavender can help reduce anxiety and promote relaxation while you breathe in the steam.

- **Eucalyptus and Tea Tree Steam**: Tea tree oil is known for its strong antimicrobial properties. Adding a few drops to your eucalyptus steam can enhance its ability to fight infections and clear the respiratory system.

Additional Benefits of Eucalyptus Steam Inhalation:

- **Helps with Dry Cough**: The moisture from the steam hydrates the respiratory tract, helping to soothe dry, irritated airways and reducing the intensity of a dry cough.

- **Supports Cold and Flu Recovery**: Eucalyptus oil's antiviral properties can support faster recovery from viral infections by helping to clear congestion and inhibit viral replication in the respiratory system.

- **Clears the Mind**: Eucalyptus oil's invigorating scent can also help improve focus and mental clarity, making it useful when you're feeling mentally foggy due to a cold or sinus infection.

Precautions:

- **Skin Sensitivity**: Essential oils are potent and should be used in small amounts. Avoid direct skin contact with undiluted eucalyptus oil, as it can cause irritation in sensitive individuals.

- **Asthma**: While eucalyptus can be beneficial for some people with asthma, it may trigger symptoms in others. Consult a healthcare provider before use if you have asthma.

- **Children**: Eucalyptus oil should be used cautiously with children, as it can be too strong for young lungs. It's advisable to consult a pediatrician before using eucalyptus oil for children under 10 years of age.

- **Pregnancy**: Pregnant women should consult with a healthcare provider before using eucalyptus essential oil for steam inhalation, as strong essential oils may not be suitable during pregnancy.

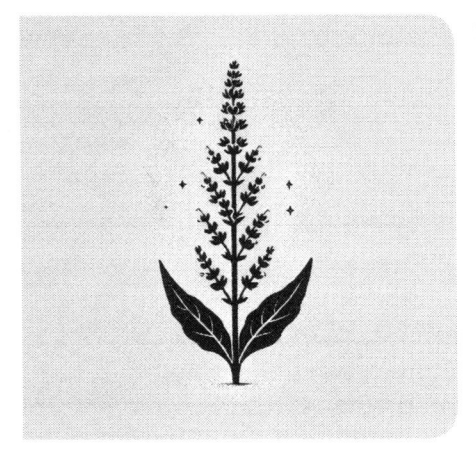

2. Mullein Lung Tea

Mullein Lung Tea is a traditional herbal remedy made from the leaves and flowers of the *Verbascum thapsus* plant, commonly known as mullein. This herb has been used for centuries to support respiratory health, especially for conditions like coughs, bronchitis, and asthma. Mullein is known for its expectorant, anti-inflammatory, and soothing properties, making it an excellent remedy for clearing mucus, calming irritated airways, and promoting lung health.

Key Benefits of Mullein Lung Tea:

- **Supports Lung Health**: Mullein acts as an expectorant, helping to loosen and expel mucus from the lungs and airways. It is particularly useful for respiratory conditions like bronchitis, asthma, and persistent coughs.

- **Reduces Inflammation in the Respiratory Tract**: Mullein contains compounds like **saponins** and **mucilage**, which soothe inflamed and irritated tissues in the lungs and throat. This helps calm conditions that cause inflammation, such as bronchitis and asthma.

- **Eases Coughs**: Mullein's soothing properties help calm dry, irritating coughs by moisturizing the respiratory tract. It also makes wet coughs more productive by helping the body expel excess mucus.

- **Relieves Asthma and Bronchitis Symptoms**: Mullein has mild bronchodilator properties, meaning it helps open the airways and makes breathing easier. This makes it helpful for people with asthma or bronchitis who experience wheezing or shortness of breath.

- **Natural Antimicrobial Properties**: Mullein has mild antimicrobial properties that help combat respiratory infections, making it useful in preventing and treating mild infections that affect the lungs and airways.

How to Make Mullein Lung Tea:

Ingredients:

- 1-2 teaspoons dried mullein leaves (or 1 mullein tea bag)
- 1 cup boiling water
- Optional: honey or lemon for added flavor and benefits

Instructions:

1. Bring water to a boil and allow it to cool slightly before pouring it over the mullein leaves or tea bag.

2. Place the dried mullein in a tea infuser or directly into a mug.

3. Pour the hot water over the mullein and let it steep for 10-15 minutes to extract its beneficial compounds.

4. Strain the tea through a fine mesh strainer or use a tea bag to avoid any tiny hairs from the mullein leaves, which may irritate the throat.

5. Add honey or lemon if desired to enhance flavor and soothe the throat.

6. Sip slowly to enjoy the lung-clearing effects of mullein.

Dosage:

- **For respiratory support**: Drink 1-2 cups of mullein tea daily to help soothe the lungs and promote respiratory health.
- **For acute conditions**: During respiratory infections, bronchitis, or asthma flare-ups, drink up to 3 cups daily to help loosen mucus and reduce inflammation.

Science Behind Mullein's Respiratory Benefits:

Mullein contains **saponins**, which act as natural expectorants, helping to break up and expel mucus from the lungs. This makes it particularly effective for clearing congestion in the respiratory tract. Additionally, the herb is rich in **mucilage**, a gel-like substance that coats and soothes irritated tissues in the throat and lungs, helping to calm dry, hacking coughs or irritation caused by inflammation.

Research published in the *Journal of Ethnopharmacology* supports mullein's use in treating respiratory conditions, noting its ability to ease symptoms of asthma, bronchitis, and other lung diseases by reducing inflammation and promoting mucus clearance. Its mild antimicrobial properties also help fight off respiratory infections, such as colds or the flu.

Variations and Additions:

- **Mullein and Licorice Root Tea**: Add licorice root for its additional soothing and anti-inflammatory properties. Licorice complements mullein's effects by further calming irritated airways and easing coughs.
- **Mullein and Peppermint Tea**: Peppermint can help clear the sinuses and add a refreshing flavor to your mullein tea. It also enhances respiratory function by acting as a mild bronchodilator, helping to open up the airways.
- **Mullein and Ginger Tea**: Ginger adds a warming effect and helps with respiratory circulation, making it a great addition to mullein tea. It also has anti-inflammatory properties that complement mullein's lung-clearing benefits.
- **Mullein and Thyme Tea**: Thyme is another herb known for its expectorant and antimicrobial properties. Combining mullein and thyme creates a potent lung-clearing tea that helps reduce mucus and combat respiratory infections.

Additional Benefits of Mullein Tea:

- **Soothes Throat Irritation**: Mullein's mucilage content helps coat the throat, reducing irritation from coughing or sore throat, especially during cold and flu season.
- **Allergy Relief**: Mullein may help reduce inflammation and congestion caused by seasonal allergies, acting as a natural remedy for allergic rhinitis or hay fever.
- **Anti-Inflammatory**: Mullein's anti-inflammatory properties not only benefit the respiratory system but can also be helpful for general inflammation in the body, offering relief from conditions like joint pain or muscle soreness.

Precautions:

Mullein tea is generally considered safe when used appropriately, but there are a few precautions to consider:

- **Avoid Tiny Hairs**: Mullein leaves have fine hairs that can irritate the throat if not strained properly. Always strain the tea through a fine mesh to avoid irritation.
- **Pregnancy and Breastfeeding**: Pregnant or breastfeeding women should consult a healthcare provider before using mullein, as its safety during pregnancy has not been well-studied.
- **Allergic Reactions**: People with sensitivities to plants in the Scrophulariaceae family should use caution when consuming mullein, as they may experience allergic reactions.

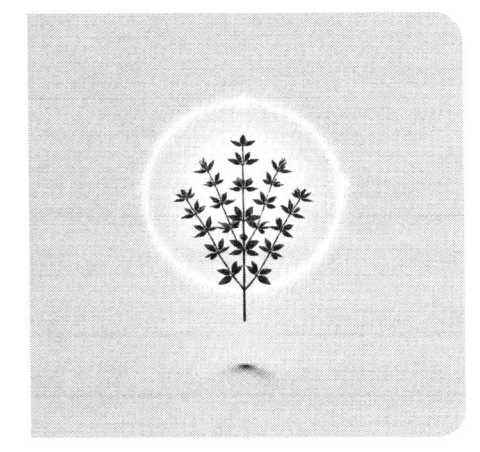

3. Thyme Cough Syrup

Thyme Cough Syrup is a natural, homemade remedy made from the leaves of the *Thymus vulgaris* plant, commonly known as thyme. Thyme has long been used in herbal medicine for its antimicrobial, expectorant, and anti-inflammatory properties, making it an effective treatment for soothing coughs, loosening mucus, and alleviating respiratory discomfort. This herbal syrup combines the potency of thyme with the soothing qualities of honey to provide relief from coughs and respiratory infections.

Key Benefits of Thyme Cough Syrup:

- **Soothes Coughs**: Thyme helps calm both dry and productive coughs by relaxing the muscles of the trachea and bronchi, reducing the frequency and severity of coughing fits.
- **Acts as an Expectorant**: Thyme's expectorant properties promote the clearance of mucus from the airways, making it easier to expel phlegm and reducing congestion, especially useful for wet or chesty coughs.
- **Antimicrobial Properties**: Thyme is rich in **thymol**, a powerful compound with antimicrobial properties that help fight off respiratory infections, including bacterial and viral infections that cause colds, bronchitis, and sore throats.
- **Reduces Inflammation**: Thyme has anti-inflammatory effects, which help soothe irritation in the respiratory tract, relieving the discomfort associated with sore throats, bronchitis, and other respiratory issues.
- **Supports Immune Function**: The combination of thyme and honey boosts the immune system, helping the body recover from infections more quickly while reducing the duration of cold symptoms.

How to Make Thyme Cough Syrup:

Ingredients:
- 1 cup fresh thyme leaves (or ½ cup dried thyme)
- 1 cup water
- 1 cup raw honey
- Optional: 1 tablespoon lemon juice (for added flavor and vitamin C)

Instructions:

1. In a small saucepan, bring the water to a boil, then reduce the heat to a simmer.
2. Add the fresh or dried thyme to the simmering water and cover the pan. Allow the thyme to steep for 15-20 minutes to fully extract its medicinal properties.
3. Remove from heat and strain the liquid through a fine mesh strainer or cheesecloth to remove the thyme leaves.
4. Once the thyme-infused water has cooled slightly (but is still warm), stir in the honey until fully dissolved. If using, add the lemon juice for an extra boost of vitamin C and flavor.
5. Pour the syrup into a clean glass jar or bottle and store it in the refrigerator. The syrup will last for about 2 weeks.

Dosage:

- **For adults**: Take 1 tablespoon of thyme syrup every 3-4 hours as needed to soothe coughs and clear mucus.
- **For children over 1 year old**: Administer 1 teaspoon every 3-4 hours. (Do not give honey to children under 1 year of age due to the risk of botulism.)

Science Behind Thyme's Benefits for Coughs:

Thyme is rich in **thymol**, a volatile compound known for its antimicrobial, antifungal, and expectorant properties. Research published in the journal *Planta Medica* found that thymol can relax the respiratory muscles, helping to open airways and ease coughing. Thyme's expectorant properties also encourage the clearance of mucus, making it an ideal herb for treating chest congestion and productive coughs.

In addition to thymol, thyme contains **carvacrol**, another potent compound that helps reduce inflammation in the respiratory tract. Together, these compounds make thyme effective for treating infections and reducing the inflammation and irritation that lead to coughing.

Honey, a key ingredient in this syrup, has been shown to be as effective as some over-the-counter cough suppressants. It works by coating and soothing the throat, reducing the irritation that triggers coughing. Honey also has natural antimicrobial properties, further aiding in the fight against infections.

Variations and Additions:

- **Thyme and Ginger Syrup**: Add a few slices of fresh ginger to the thyme infusion for additional anti-inflammatory and soothing benefits. Ginger helps relieve respiratory inflammation and ease coughing.
- **Thyme and Licorice Root Syrup**: Licorice root is a natural demulcent that soothes the throat and reduces coughing. Adding licorice root to your thyme syrup will provide extra relief for dry, irritated throats.
- **Thyme and Echinacea Syrup**: Echinacea can be added to the syrup to enhance immune support, especially during cold and flu season, helping the body fend off infections.
- **Thyme and Peppermint Syrup**: Add peppermint leaves for a cooling effect that helps clear nasal congestion and soothe inflamed airways.

Additional Benefits of Thyme Cough Syrup:

- **Relieves Sore Throat**: The combination of thyme and honey soothes sore throats by reducing inflammation and coating the mucous membranes, providing relief from irritation.
- **Antioxidant Protection**: Both thyme and honey are rich in antioxidants, which help protect the body from oxidative stress and support immune health during respiratory infections.
- **Safe and Natural**: Thyme cough syrup offers a natural alternative to over-the-counter cough medicines, free of artificial additives and chemicals, making it gentle yet effective for both adults and children (over 1 year old).

Precautions:

- **Not for Infants**: Do not give honey to children under 1 year of age due to the risk of infant botulism.
- **Thyme Allergies**: Individuals who are allergic to plants in the mint family (*Lamiaceae*), which includes thyme, should avoid using thyme-based remedies.
- **Pregnancy and Breastfeeding**: While thyme is generally considered safe in food amounts, pregnant or breastfeeding women should consult a healthcare provider before using thyme in medicinal doses.
- **Asthma**: While thyme can be helpful for respiratory issues, some individuals with asthma may find that certain herbs trigger their symptoms. It's advisable to consult with a healthcare provider if you have asthma and are considering using thyme for respiratory relief.

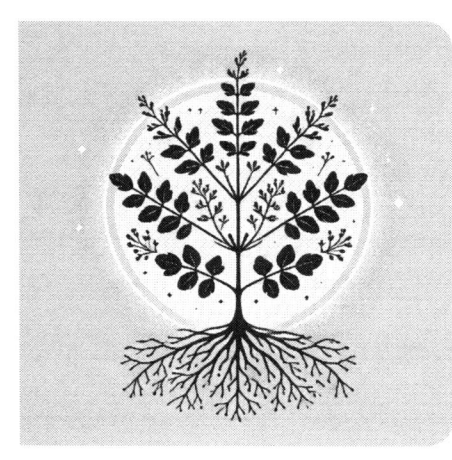

4. Licorice Root Respiratory Tonic

Licorice Root Respiratory Tonic is a soothing herbal remedy made from the root of the *Glycyrrhiza glabra* plant, which has been used for centuries in traditional medicine to support respiratory health. Licorice root is renowned for its ability to soothe the throat, reduce inflammation, and promote mucus production, making it especially beneficial for respiratory conditions such as bronchitis, asthma, and coughs. Its anti-inflammatory, expectorant, and immune-boosting properties make it an excellent remedy for a range of respiratory ailments.

Key Benefits of Licorice Root Respiratory Tonic:

- **Soothes the Throat and Airway Irritation**: Licorice root contains **mucilage**, a gel-like substance that coats and soothes the mucous membranes in the respiratory tract. This helps alleviate throat irritation and calm dry, scratchy coughs.
- **Reduces Inflammation**: Licorice root is rich in **glycyrrhizin**, a compound with strong anti-inflammatory properties. This helps reduce inflammation in the airways, providing relief from conditions like asthma, bronchitis, and sore throats.
- **Acts as an Expectorant**: Licorice root promotes the production of healthy mucus, which helps clear phlegm and congestion from the lungs. This makes it especially helpful for productive coughs, allowing the body to expel mucus more effectively.
- **Boosts Immune Function**: Licorice root has immune-enhancing properties that help the body fight off respiratory infections, such as colds, flu, and bronchitis. It stimulates the production of interferon, a protein that helps combat viral infections.
- **Supports Adrenal Health**: Licorice root helps regulate cortisol levels and support adrenal function, making it helpful for those dealing with respiratory issues linked to stress or weakened immunity.

How to Make Licorice Root Respiratory Tonic:

Ingredients:
- 1 tablespoon dried licorice root (organic)
- 2 cups water
- 1 teaspoon honey (optional, for added soothing and sweetness)
- Optional: ½ teaspoon cinnamon or fresh ginger (for extra warming and anti-inflammatory benefits)

Instructions:

1. After In a small saucepan, combine the licorice root and water.
2. Bring the mixture to a boil, then reduce the heat and let it simmer for 10-15 minutes to fully extract the licorice root's beneficial compounds.
3. Remove from heat and let the tonic cool slightly. Strain the mixture through a fine mesh strainer to remove the licorice root.
4. Stir in honey if desired for added sweetness and throat-soothing properties. You can also add a pinch of cinnamon or fresh ginger for extra flavor and benefits.
5. Pour the tonic into a cup and sip slowly, allowing the licorice root to soothe your respiratory system.

Dosage:

- **For respiratory support**: Drink 1 cup of licorice root tonic 1-2 times daily to relieve coughs, soothe throat irritation, and reduce airway inflammation.
- **For acute conditions**: During respiratory infections or flare-ups of conditions like bronchitis or asthma, drink up to 3 cups per day for enhanced relief.

Science Behind Licorice Root's Benefits for Respiratory Health:

Licorice root's active compound, **glycyrrhizin**, has been extensively studied for its anti-inflammatory, antimicrobial, and immune-boosting effects. Glycyrrhizin reduces inflammation by inhibiting the release of inflammatory cytokines and prostaglandins, making it particularly effective for conditions like asthma and bronchitis, where airway inflammation is a major issue. Additionally, glycyrrhizin promotes the production of protective mucus in the respiratory tract, helping to loosen phlegm and make coughs more productive.

Research published in the *Journal of Ethnopharmacology* has shown that licorice root has expectorant properties, helping to clear excess mucus from the lungs. Studies have also highlighted its antiviral activity, which is beneficial for preventing and treating respiratory infections, such as colds and the flu.

Variations and Additions:

- **Licorice Root and Ginger Tonic**: Add fresh ginger slices to the licorice root tonic for an extra warming and anti-inflammatory effect. Ginger helps improve circulation and supports the respiratory system, especially during colds or bronchitis.
- **Licorice Root and Marshmallow Root Tonic**: Combine licorice root with marshmallow root for additional soothing of the throat and lungs. Both herbs contain mucilage, which coats the respiratory tract and eases irritation from persistent coughing.
- **Licorice Root and Thyme Tonic**: Thyme has powerful antimicrobial and expectorant properties. Adding it to licorice root tonic enhances the ability to clear mucus and fight off respiratory infections.
- **Licorice Root and Peppermint Tonic**: Add peppermint for a refreshing, cooling effect that helps open up the airways and reduce congestion, making breathing easier, especially during colds or sinus congestion.

Additional Benefits of Licorice Root:

- **Supports Digestive Health**: Licorice root also soothes digestive issues such as indigestion, heartburn, and ulcers by reducing inflammation in the stomach lining.
- **Hormonal Balance**: Licorice root helps balance cortisol levels and support adrenal function, which is especially beneficial for individuals dealing with stress-related respiratory issues.
- **Antioxidant Protection**: Licorice root is rich in flavonoids and antioxidants that protect the body from oxidative stress, reducing the overall inflammatory response.

Precautions:

- **Glycyrrhizin Content**: While licorice root is beneficial, it should be used in moderation due to its glycyrrhizin content, which can lead to elevated blood pressure, low potassium levels, and water retention in some individuals if consumed in excessive amounts.
- **Pregnancy and Breastfeeding**: Pregnant and breastfeeding women should avoid using licorice root in large amounts, as it may affect hormone levels or cause uterine stimulation.
- **Health Conditions**: People with high blood pressure, kidney disease, or heart conditions should consult a healthcare provider before using licorice root, as its glycyrrhizin content can exacerbate these conditions.
- **Medication Interactions**: Licorice root may interact with certain medications, including blood pressure medications and corticosteroids. Always consult a healthcare provider before using licorice root if you are on medication.

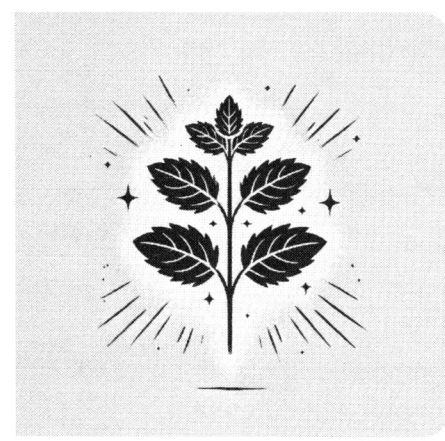

5. Peppermint Chest Balm

Peppermint Chest Balm is a soothing topical remedy made from peppermint essential oil and other natural ingredients designed to relieve congestion, ease breathing, and reduce discomfort associated with respiratory conditions like colds, bronchitis, and sinus congestion. Peppermint is rich in **menthol**, which has cooling, decongestant, and anti-inflammatory properties. When applied to the chest, this balm provides a refreshing sensation that helps open the airways, clear nasal passages, and reduce coughing.

Key Benefits of Peppermint Chest Balm:

- **Decongests the Sinuses and Chest**: Peppermint's active compound, **menthol**, acts as a natural decongestant by helping to clear mucus and open the nasal passages, making breathing easier during colds, sinus infections, or allergies.
- **Relieves Coughs and Throat Irritation**: The cooling effect of menthol soothes irritation in the throat and respiratory tract, helping to calm persistent coughs and ease discomfort from chest tightness or inflammation.
- **Reduces Inflammation**: Peppermint has anti-inflammatory properties that help calm inflamed airways and soothe bronchial irritation, making it beneficial for conditions like bronchitis and asthma.
- **Promotes Relaxation and Sleep**: The invigorating yet calming scent of peppermint helps relax the body and mind, promoting deeper breathing and aiding relaxation, which can be especially helpful for nighttime congestion and discomfort.
- **Natural Pain Reliever**: Peppermint oil can also reduce muscle soreness and chest tightness by relaxing muscles and reducing pain. Its mild analgesic properties make it helpful for relieving aches and tension in the chest area during respiratory illnesses.

How to Make Peppermint Chest Balm:

Ingredients:
- 1/4 cup coconut oil (or olive oil)
- 2 tablespoons beeswax (for thickening)
- 10-15 drops peppermint essential oil
- 5-10 drops eucalyptus essential oil (optional, for added decongestant power)
- 5 drops lavender essential oil (optional, for calming effects)

Instructions:

1. In a double boiler, melt the coconut oil and beeswax together over low heat until fully liquified. Stir well to combine.
2. Remove the mixture from heat and allow it to cool slightly for 1-2 minutes.
3. Stir in the peppermint essential oil, and if using, add the eucalyptus and lavender essential oils for enhanced benefits.
4. Pour the mixture into a clean, airtight jar or tin and let it cool and solidify at room temperature (this may take 1-2 hours).
5. Once solidified, your peppermint chest balm is ready to use. Store it in a cool, dry place, and it will last for several months.

How to Use:

- **For congestion relief**: Apply a small amount of the balm to your chest, throat, and back, massaging gently to allow the essential oils to absorb into the skin. The menthol will create a cooling sensation that helps clear the airways and reduce congestion.
- **For coughs and chest discomfort**: Apply before bed or during the day to calm coughing and ease chest tightness. The soothing scent and properties of the balm can also help promote restful sleep.

Science Behind Peppermint's Respiratory Benefits:

Peppermint's main active compound, **menthol**, is well-known for its decongestant and antitussive (cough-suppressing) effects. Menthol triggers cold-sensitive receptors in the nose and throat, creating a cooling sensation that helps open the airways and reduce the feeling of congestion. Studies published in the *Journal of Pharmacognosy and Phytochemistry* have shown that inhaling menthol can improve nasal airflow, making it easier to breathe, especially during respiratory illnesses like colds or bronchitis.

Peppermint oil also has mild **anti-inflammatory** and **antimicrobial** properties, which help reduce inflammation in the airways and fight off bacteria or viruses that can cause respiratory infections. The addition of **eucalyptus oil** in the balm enhances these effects, as eucalyptus is another potent decongestant and anti-inflammatory agent used in respiratory care.

Variations and Additions:

- **Peppermint and Eucalyptus Chest Balm**: Add 10-15 drops of eucalyptus essential oil to boost the decongestant and expectorant properties of the balm. Eucalyptus is highly effective for opening airways and clearing mucus.
- **Peppermint and Lavender Chest Balm**: Adding lavender oil creates a calming and soothing balm that helps reduce anxiety and promote better sleep, especially for children or those with difficulty sleeping due to congestion.
- **Peppermint and Ginger Chest Balm**: Ginger oil adds a warming effect to the balm, helping to relieve chest tightness and muscle aches caused by coughing or respiratory infections.
- **Peppermint Vapor Rub**: For an even more powerful decongestant balm, increase the peppermint oil and add a few drops of camphor oil, which is often found in over-the-counter vapor rubs for its ability to clear sinuses and reduce chest discomfort.

Additional Benefits of Peppermint Chest Balm:

- **Soothes Headaches**: Rubbing a small amount of peppermint balm on the temples or the back of the neck can help alleviate tension headaches or sinus headaches, especially those caused by congestion.
- **Reduces Muscle Aches**: The cooling and analgesic properties of peppermint oil make this balm useful for massaging sore muscles or relieving body aches that often accompany colds or flu.
- **Natural Insect Repellent**: Peppermint oil is also known for its insect-repellent properties, so the balm can help keep mosquitoes and other bugs at bay when applied to the skin.

Precautions:

- **Skin Sensitivity**: Essential oils, especially peppermint and eucalyptus, can be strong and may cause irritation in sensitive individuals. Always perform a patch test on a small area of skin before widespread use, and dilute the balm further if irritation occurs.
- **Children**: Peppermint oil may be too strong for young children, particularly infants and toddlers. For children under 5, consult with a healthcare provider before using peppermint oil on the skin, or consider using milder essential oils like lavender or chamomile.
- **Avoid Contact with Eyes and Mucous Membranes**: When applying the balm, avoid getting it near the eyes or inside the nose, as menthol and essential oils can cause irritation.
- **Pregnancy and Breastfeeding**: Pregnant and breastfeeding women should consult with a healthcare provider before using essential oils topically, especially in medicinal doses.

Chapter 6

Promoting Cardiovascular Wellness

- The Importance of Heart Health
- Top 5 Herbal Recipes for a Healthy Heart
  1. Hawthorn Berry Heart Tonic
  2. Garlic and Olive Oil Spread
  3. Ginkgo Biloba Circulation Tea
  4. Motherwort Heart Support
  5. Turmeric Anti-Inflammatory Latte

The Importance of Heart Health

The Importance of Heart Health cannot be overstated, as the heart is the engine of the body, responsible for pumping oxygen-rich blood and essential nutrients to every organ and tissue. Maintaining a healthy heart is essential for overall well-being and longevity, as heart-related diseases, including coronary artery disease, heart attacks, and heart failure, remain the leading causes of death worldwide. Promoting heart health involves a combination of lifestyle factors such as diet, physical activity, stress management, and regular medical care. Understanding the role the heart plays in the body and the factors that influence its function is key to preventing cardiovascular diseases and improving quality of life.

The Role of the Heart:

The heart is a muscular organ that works tirelessly to keep the circulatory system functioning. It pumps blood through a network of arteries, veins, and capillaries, delivering oxygen and nutrients while removing waste products like carbon dioxide. The heart typically beats around 100,000 times a day, supplying the body with the oxygen and fuel it needs to function properly.

The heart has four chambers – two atria and two ventricles – that work in coordination to ensure that oxygen-poor blood is sent to the lungs for oxygenation and that oxygen-rich blood is circulated throughout the body. The heart also plays a critical role in maintaining blood pressure, controlling blood flow, and ensuring that all parts of the body are adequately nourished.

Common Heart Diseases and Conditions:

1. **Coronary Artery Disease (CAD):** This occurs when the arteries supplying blood to the heart become narrowed or blocked due to a buildup of plaque (atherosclerosis). CAD can lead to chest pain (angina) or heart attacks.

2. **Heart Attack (Myocardial Infarction):** A heart attack occurs when blood flow to part of the heart muscle is blocked, often due to a clot in one of the coronary arteries. Without prompt treatment, the affected part of the heart muscle can be permanently damaged.

3. **Congestive Heart Failure:** This is a condition in which the heart cannot pump blood efficiently, leading to fluid buildup in the lungs and other tissues. Symptoms include shortness of breath, fatigue, and swelling in the legs.

4. **Arrhythmias:** These are irregular heartbeats, which can be harmless or life-threatening. Common types include atrial fibrillation, tachycardia, and bradycardia, where the heart beats too fast, too slow, or irregularly.

5. **High Blood Pressure (Hypertension):** Often called the "silent killer" because it typically has no symptoms, hypertension can damage the heart and blood vessels over time, increasing the risk of heart attack, stroke, and kidney disease.

6. **Cardiomyopathy:** This refers to diseases of the heart muscle that can affect the heart's ability to pump blood effectively, leading to heart failure or arrhythmias.

86. Ch. 5 - Promoting Cardiovascular Wellness

Factors Influencing Heart Health:

- **Diet**: What you eat has a direct impact on your heart. A diet rich in fruits, vegetables, whole grains, lean proteins, and healthy fats (such as omega-3 fatty acids) supports heart health. In contrast, diets high in saturated fats, trans fats, sodium, and refined sugars contribute to the buildup of plaque in the arteries, raising the risk of heart disease.

- **Physical Activity**: Regular physical activity strengthens the heart muscle, improves circulation, and helps regulate blood pressure and cholesterol levels. Even moderate exercise, like walking or cycling, can significantly reduce the risk of cardiovascular disease.

- **Weight Management**: Being overweight or obese puts extra strain on the heart and increases the likelihood of developing conditions like high blood pressure, diabetes, and high cholesterol, all of which raise the risk of heart disease.

- **Cholesterol Levels**: High levels of LDL (low-density lipoprotein) cholesterol, often referred to as "bad cholesterol," can lead to plaque buildup in the arteries, while HDL (high-density lipoprotein) or "good cholesterol" helps remove cholesterol from the bloodstream.

- **Blood Pressure**: Keeping blood pressure within a healthy range (below 120/80 mmHg) is crucial for preventing damage to the heart and arteries. Hypertension increases the risk of heart attacks and strokes.

- **Smoking**: Tobacco use is one of the most significant risk factors for heart disease. Smoking damages the lining of the arteries, leading to plaque buildup, and reduces the amount of oxygen in the blood, forcing the heart to work harder.

- **Stress**: Chronic stress can negatively affect heart health by raising blood pressure, triggering unhealthy habits (such as overeating or smoking), and increasing inflammation in the body. Learning to manage stress through relaxation techniques, mindfulness, or exercise is vital for heart health.

- **Sleep**: Poor sleep, especially conditions like sleep apnea, has been linked to an increased risk of heart disease, as it can lead to high blood pressure, obesity, and insulin resistance.

The Importance of Heart Health for Longevity:

Maintaining heart health is key to living a long and active life. Cardiovascular diseases are a leading cause of disability and reduced quality of life, particularly in older adults. Taking preventive measures to protect the heart can delay or prevent the onset of heart-related diseases, reduce the need for medication or surgery, and improve overall well-being. Healthy heart function ensures that all body systems receive the oxygen and nutrients they need to thrive, which in turn supports mental clarity, physical endurance, and emotional stability.

Steps to Improve and Maintain Heart Health:

1. **Eat a Heart-Healthy Diet**: Incorporate more fruits, vegetables, whole grains, and lean proteins, while reducing salt, sugar, and unhealthy fats. The Mediterranean diet, rich in olive oil, fish, nuts, and whole grains, has been shown to reduce heart disease risk.

2. **Exercise Regularly**: Aim for at least 150 minutes of moderate aerobic activity, such as brisk walking, or 75 minutes of vigorous activity, like running, each week. Strength training also benefits the heart by improving muscle mass and metabolism.

3. **Monitor Cholesterol and Blood Pressure**: Regular health checkups can help monitor and manage cholesterol levels and blood pressure, reducing the risk of heart attacks and strokes.

4. **Quit Smoking**: If you smoke, quitting is one of the best things you can do for your heart. The risk of heart disease starts to decrease soon after quitting, and within a few years, the risk is comparable to that of a non-smoker.

5. **Manage Stress**: Incorporating stress-relief practices like yoga, meditation, deep breathing, and hobbies that promote relaxation can help keep stress levels in check, reducing the negative effects on the heart.

6. **Get Quality Sleep**: Aim for 7-9 hours of quality sleep each night. Poor sleep, particularly from conditions like sleep apnea, can lead to higher risks of heart problems.

7. **Limit Alcohol**: Excessive alcohol consumption can lead to high blood pressure, arrhythmias, and heart failure. Moderate drinking, defined as up to one drink per day for women and two drinks per day for men, is key.

8. **Maintain a Healthy Weight**: Managing weight through a healthy diet and regular exercise reduces the strain on the heart and decreases the risk of developing high blood pressure and diabetes.

Top 5 Herbal Recipes for a Healthy Heart

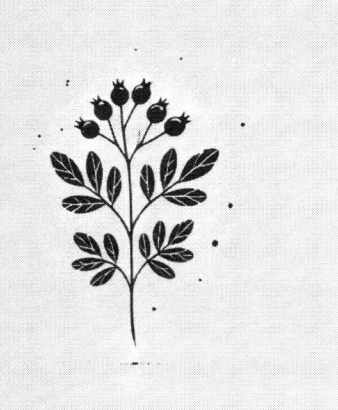

1. Hawthorn Berry Heart Tonic

Hawthorn Berry Heart Tonic is a traditional herbal remedy made from the berries of the *Crataegus* plant, commonly known as hawthorn. This powerful heart tonic has been used for centuries to strengthen and protect the cardiovascular system. Hawthorn berries are rich in antioxidants, including flavonoids, which have been shown to improve heart function, lower blood pressure, enhance circulation, and reduce inflammation. This tonic is especially beneficial for individuals with mild to moderate heart conditions, such as high blood pressure, angina, or heart failure, and for those looking to maintain overall heart health.

Key Benefits of Hawthorn Berry Heart Tonic:

- **Strengthens Heart Function**: Hawthorn is known to improve the contractility of the heart, helping it pump more efficiently. It is particularly beneficial for individuals with weakened heart muscles, as it enhances the heart's ability to circulate blood effectively.

- **Lowers Blood Pressure**: Hawthorn berries help dilate blood vessels, which improves blood flow and reduces blood pressure. This makes it a natural remedy for hypertension and for preventing strain on the heart and blood vessels.

- **Improves Circulation**: By enhancing the flow of blood through the arteries and veins, hawthorn helps ensure that the heart, brain, and other organs receive adequate oxygen and nutrients. This is particularly helpful for people with circulatory issues or those recovering from heart conditions.

- **Reduces Angina and Chest Pain**: Hawthorn's vasodilating properties help increase blood flow to the heart, reducing the frequency and severity of chest pain (angina) caused by restricted blood flow.

- **Rich in Antioxidants**: Hawthorn berries are high in flavonoids and procyanidins, which protect the heart by neutralizing free radicals that can damage blood vessels and the heart muscle. This helps prevent the progression of heart disease.

- **Balances Cholesterol**: Hawthorn has been shown to help lower LDL ("bad") cholesterol levels while promoting the production of HDL ("good") cholesterol, further supporting cardiovascular health by reducing plaque buildup in the arteries.

How to Make Hawthorn Berry Heart Tonic:

Ingredients:

- 1 cup dried hawthorn berries (or 2 cups fresh berries)
- 4 cups water
- 1 tablespoon honey (optional, for added sweetness and heart-soothing properties)
- Optional: 1 cinnamon stick or 1 tablespoon dried hibiscus flowers (for added flavor and cardiovascular support)

Instructions:

1. In a medium saucepan, combine the dried hawthorn berries and water.

2. Bring the mixture to a boil, then reduce the heat and let it simmer for 30-40 minutes to extract the medicinal compounds from the berries.

3. Remove from heat and let the mixture cool slightly. Strain the liquid through a fine mesh strainer or cheesecloth, pressing the berries to extract as much liquid as possible.

4. If desired, stir in the honey for added flavor and sweetness. You can also add a cinnamon

stick or hibiscus during the simmering process for additional heart-health benefits and a rich, tangy flavor.

5. Pour the tonic into a clean glass jar or bottle and store it in the refrigerator for up to a week.

Dosage:

- **For heart health maintenance**: Drink 1-2 tablespoons of the tonic daily, diluted in water or tea.
- **For cardiovascular support**: Take 1-2 tablespoons 2-3 times a day to help manage blood pressure, improve circulation, and support overall heart function.

Science Behind Hawthorn's Benefits for Heart Health:

Hawthorn berries contain potent **flavonoids** like **quercetin**, **vitexin**, and **procyanidins**, which have been extensively studied for their cardioprotective effects. These compounds help improve blood flow to the heart, increase the strength of heart contractions, and reduce resistance in the blood vessels, lowering blood pressure. Studies published in the *Journal of the American College of Cardiology* have shown that hawthorn can improve symptoms in people with chronic heart failure by enhancing cardiac output and reducing fatigue and shortness of breath.

Hawthorn also has mild **diuretic** properties, which help reduce fluid retention and swelling in people with heart failure, alleviating the strain on the heart. The high antioxidant content of hawthorn berries protects the blood vessels from oxidative stress, preventing damage that can lead to atherosclerosis (hardening of the arteries).

Variations and Additions:

- **Hawthorn and Hibiscus Heart Tonic**: Add dried hibiscus flowers to the tonic for additional heart support. Hibiscus is known to help lower blood pressure and is rich in antioxidants that support cardiovascular health.
- **Hawthorn and Ginger Heart Tonic**: Ginger's warming and anti-inflammatory properties can enhance circulation and improve the heart's function. Add fresh ginger slices to the tonic for extra cardiovascular support.
- **Hawthorn and Lemon Balm Tonic**: Lemon balm has calming properties that reduce stress and anxiety, which can also benefit the heart by lowering blood pressure and heart rate. This combination is especially useful for stress-related heart conditions.
- **Hawthorn and Garlic Tonic**: Garlic is a powerful heart-healthy herb that helps lower cholesterol and blood pressure. Adding garlic to hawthorn tonic creates a potent blend for cardiovascular health.

Additional Benefits of Hawthorn Berry:

- **Reduces Anxiety and Stress**: Hawthorn has mild sedative properties, which can help reduce anxiety and stress levels. Since chronic stress negatively affects heart health by increasing blood pressure and heart rate, hawthorn can play a role in stress-related heart conditions.
- **Supports Digestion**: Hawthorn also supports digestive health by improving circulation to the digestive organs, which can help with nutrient absorption and relieve digestive discomfort.
- **Boosts Immune Function**: The antioxidants in hawthorn berries support immune health by protecting cells from damage, helping the body fight off infections more effectively.

Precautions:

- **Medication Interactions**: Hawthorn may interact with certain heart medications, including blood pressure medications, beta-blockers, and anticoagulants. If you are taking prescription medications for heart conditions, consult your healthcare provider before using hawthorn.
- **Pregnancy and Breastfeeding**: Pregnant and breastfeeding women should consult a healthcare provider before using hawthorn in medicinal doses.
- **Low Blood Pressure**: If you have low blood pressure, use hawthorn with caution, as it can lower blood pressure further.

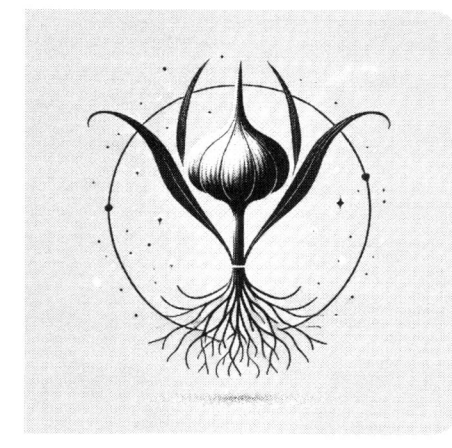

2. Garlic and Olive Oil Spread

Garlic and Olive Oil Spread is a traditional Mediterranean remedy that combines the health-boosting properties of garlic with the nourishing benefits of extra virgin olive oil. This spread has been used for centuries not only to enhance the flavor of meals but also to support cardiovascular health, boost the immune system, and reduce inflammation. Garlic contains allicin, a powerful compound known for lowering blood pressure, improving cholesterol levels, and providing antimicrobial protection. Olive oil, rich in healthy monounsaturated fats and antioxidants like polyphenols, complements garlic's benefits by supporting heart health, reducing inflammation, and improving digestion. Together, they form a potent, natural remedy for overall well-being.

Key Benefits of Garlic and Olive Oil Spread:

- **Supports Cardiovascular Health:** Garlic helps lower LDL cholesterol and blood pressure, while olive oil's healthy fats improve circulation and reduce inflammation. This combination is especially beneficial for those looking to protect against heart disease.

- **Boosts Immune Function:** Garlic's natural antimicrobial properties help fight off infections, while the antioxidants in olive oil strengthen the immune system by neutralizing free radicals.

- **Reduces Inflammation:** Both garlic and olive oil contain anti-inflammatory compounds that help alleviate chronic inflammation, which is linked to conditions such as arthritis and cardiovascular disease.

- **Enhances Digestion:** Olive oil aids in fat absorption, and garlic stimulates digestive enzymes, making this spread beneficial for digestive health and reducing bloating.

- **Rich in Antioxidants:** Olive oil is a rich source of antioxidants like vitamin E and polyphenols, while garlic provides sulfur compounds that protect cells from oxidative stress.

- **Lowers Cholesterol:** Garlic helps reduce LDL ("bad") cholesterol and may increase HDL ("good") cholesterol, while olive oil supports a healthy lipid profile, making this spread a natural choice for managing cholesterol levels.

How to Make Garlic and Olive Oil Spread:

Ingredients:
- 6 fresh garlic cloves
- ½ cup extra virgin olive oil
- Pinch of sea salt (optional)
- Optional: Fresh herbs like parsley or oregano for additional flavor and health benefits

Instructions:

1. Peel and finely mince the garlic cloves, or use a garlic press for a smoother texture.

2. In a small bowl, combine the minced garlic with olive oil, stirring to mix evenly.

3. Add a pinch of sea salt and, if desired, fresh herbs like parsley or oregano for added flavor and antioxidants.

4. Let the mixture sit for 15-20 minutes to allow the flavors to meld. For a creamier consistency, you can blend the mixture.

5. Store the spread in a sealed glass jar in the refrigerator for up to one week.

Dosage:

- For general health: Spread 1-2 teaspoons on toast or as a condiment in meals daily.
- For cardiovascular support: Take 1-2 teaspoons twice a day, mixed into salads or as a topping for vegetables.

Science Behind Garlic and Olive Oil's Benefits:

Garlic's main active compound, allicin, is responsible for many of its health benefits, including its ability to lower blood pressure, improve cholesterol levels, and fight infections. Allicin is most potent when garlic is crushed or minced. Olive oil, particularly extra virgin olive oil, is rich in monounsaturated fats and polyphenols, which have been shown to reduce inflammation, support heart health, and improve digestion. Research published in *The Journal of Nutrition* highlights the cardioprotective effects of olive oil, while studies in *Phytomedicine* confirm garlic's ability to lower blood pressure and cholesterol.

Variations and Additions:

- **Garlic and Lemon Spread:** Adding a squeeze of fresh lemon juice provides extra vitamin C and a tangy flavor that complements the spread.
- **Garlic, Olive Oil, and Chili Spread:** For a spicy kick, mix in chili flakes or fresh chili, which also adds anti-inflammatory properties.
- **Garlic and Turmeric Spread:** A pinch of turmeric can enhance the anti-inflammatory effects of the spread, especially for those with joint pain or arthritis.
- **Garlic, Olive Oil, and Basil Spread:** Fresh basil adds a fragrant aroma and boosts the antioxidant content of the spread.

Additional Benefits of Garlic and Olive Oil Spread:

- **Supports Weight Management:** Olive oil helps regulate blood sugar and reduce inflammation, aiding in weight management, while garlic can support metabolism.
- **Improves Skin Health:** The antioxidants in olive oil and garlic promote healthy skin by reducing oxidative damage and slowing the aging process.
- **Fights Respiratory Infections:** Garlic's antimicrobial and antiviral properties make this spread beneficial during cold and flu season, supporting respiratory health.

Precautions:

- **Blood-Thinning Properties:** Garlic can act as a natural blood thinner. Those on anticoagulant medications should consult their healthcare provider before consuming large amounts of garlic.
- **Allergies and Sensitivities:** Some people may experience digestive discomfort from raw garlic. Start with small amounts and adjust according to tolerance.
- **Pregnancy and Breastfeeding:** While garlic is generally safe in culinary amounts, pregnant or breastfeeding women should consult their healthcare provider before using it in large medicinal doses.

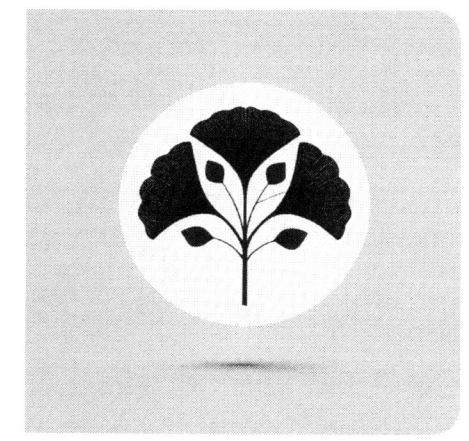

3. Ginkgo Biloba Circulation Tea

Ginkgo Biloba Circulation Tea is a traditional herbal remedy made from the leaves of the Ginkgo biloba tree, one of the oldest living tree species on Earth. This tea has been used for centuries in traditional Chinese medicine to improve circulation, support brain function, and promote overall vitality. Ginkgo leaves contain potent flavonoids and terpenoids, which are known for their ability to enhance blood flow and provide antioxidant protection. This makes Ginkgo Biloba Circulation Tea particularly beneficial for individuals with circulation issues, cognitive decline, or those seeking to maintain optimal brain and heart health.

Key Benefits of Ginkgo Biloba Circulation Tea:

- **Improves Circulation:** Ginkgo biloba helps to dilate blood vessels and increase blood flow, particularly to the brain and extremities. This makes it a useful remedy for people with poor circulation, cold hands and feet, or those suffering from conditions like peripheral artery disease.

- **Enhances Brain Function:** Ginkgo is well-known for its cognitive benefits, as it increases blood flow to the brain, potentially improving memory, focus, and mental clarity. It is often used to help manage symptoms of cognitive decline, including age-related memory issues and early-stage dementia.

- **Rich in Antioxidants:** Ginkgo leaves are high in flavonoids and terpenoids, powerful antioxidants that help neutralize free radicals and protect cells from oxidative damage. This antioxidant activity supports overall health and slows the aging process.

- **Reduces Inflammation:** The anti-inflammatory properties of Ginkgo biloba can help reduce inflammation throughout the body, making it beneficial for individuals with chronic inflammatory conditions, such as arthritis or heart disease.

- **Supports Eye Health:** By improving circulation to the eyes, Ginkgo biloba may help protect against age-related macular degeneration and other vision problems linked to poor blood flow.

How to Make Ginkgo Biloba Circulation Tea:

Ingredients:
- 1 tablespoon dried Ginkgo biloba leaves (or 2 tablespoons fresh leaves)
- 2 cups water
- Optional: 1 teaspoon honey or a slice of lemon for added flavor

Instructions:

1. Bring the water to a boil in a small saucepan.
2. Add the dried or fresh Ginkgo biloba leaves to the boiling water.
3. Reduce the heat and let the leaves simmer for 10-15 minutes to extract the medicinal compounds.
4. Remove from heat and let the tea steep for an additional 5 minutes.
5. Strain the tea into a cup, discarding the leaves. If desired, add honey or lemon to enhance the flavor.
6. Enjoy the tea while warm, and store any leftovers in the refrigerator for up to two days.

Dosage:

- For general circulation support: Drink 1 cup of Ginkgo biloba tea daily.
- For cognitive or circulatory benefits: Drink 1-2 cups of tea daily, as needed.

Science Behind Ginkgo Biloba's Benefits for Circulation:

Ginkgo biloba improves circulation by dilating blood vessels and reducing platelet aggregation, which helps to improve blood flow and reduce the risk of blood clots. Studies have shown that Ginkgo biloba can improve blood flow to the brain and extremities, which is particularly beneficial for individuals with poor circulation or cognitive decline. In addition to its circulatory benefits, Ginkgo is rich in antioxidants that protect cells from oxidative stress. Research published in *Phytomedicine* has demonstrated Ginkgo's potential in improving cognitive function in older adults and protecting against neurodegenerative diseases like Alzheimer's.

Variations and Additions:

- **Ginkgo and Ginseng Tea:** Ginseng is another potent herbal remedy for circulation and energy. Combining Ginkgo with ginseng can enhance stamina and support cardiovascular health.
- **Ginkgo and Ginger Circulation Tea:** Ginger's warming and anti-inflammatory properties complement Ginkgo's ability to improve blood flow. This combination is particularly helpful for individuals with cold extremities or joint pain.
- **Ginkgo and Lemon Balm Tea:** Lemon balm has calming properties that help reduce stress and anxiety. Combining it with Ginkgo can support cognitive function while promoting relaxation and stress relief.
- **Ginkgo and Hawthorn Tea:** Hawthorn is another powerful cardiovascular herb. Together with Ginkgo, it can further support circulation and heart health.

Additional Benefits of Ginkgo Biloba:

- **Supports Mental Clarity:** Ginkgo's ability to enhance blood flow to the brain may improve memory and focus, making it a popular choice for students and those who need mental clarity.
- **May Help with Anxiety:** Some studies suggest that Ginkgo biloba can help reduce symptoms of anxiety, likely due to its ability to enhance blood flow and balance stress hormones.
- **Protects Against Neurodegenerative Diseases:** Ginkgo's antioxidant and anti-inflammatory properties make it a potential protective agent against conditions like Alzheimer's and Parkinson's disease.
- **Promotes Skin Health:** By improving circulation and delivering more nutrients to the skin, Ginkgo can help improve skin elasticity and reduce the appearance of wrinkles and fine lines.

Precautions:

- **Medication Interactions:** Ginkgo biloba may interact with certain medications, including blood thinners, anticoagulants, and antiplatelet drugs. Consult your healthcare provider before using Ginkgo if you are on these medications.
- **Surgery:** If you are scheduled for surgery, discontinue Ginkgo at least two weeks before, as it can increase the risk of bleeding.
- **Pregnancy and Breastfeeding:** Pregnant and breastfeeding women should consult a healthcare provider before using Ginkgo biloba in medicinal doses.
- **Headaches or Dizziness:** Some individuals may experience mild side effects like headaches, dizziness, or gastrointestinal discomfort when using Ginkgo. If these symptoms occur, reduce the dosage or discontinue use.

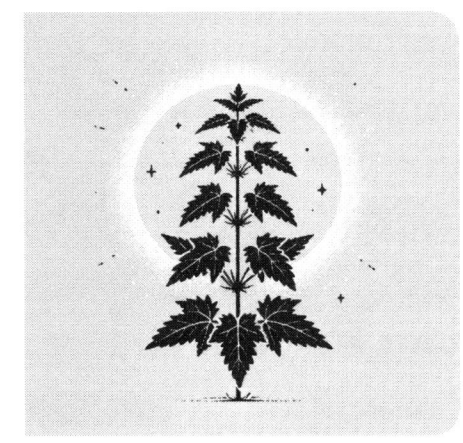

4. Motherwort Heart Support

Motherwort Heart Support is a traditional herbal remedy made from the leaves and flowers of *Leonurus cardiaca*, commonly known as motherwort. This herb has been used for centuries to support heart health, particularly in easing heart palpitations, reducing anxiety, and promoting overall cardiovascular function. Motherwort is rich in alkaloids, flavonoids, and iridoids that help strengthen the heart muscle, regulate heartbeat, and calm the nervous system. It is especially beneficial for individuals with mild heart conditions, stress-related heart issues, or those looking to maintain heart health naturally.

Key Benefits of Motherwort Heart Support:

- **Regulates Heartbeat:** Motherwort is known to help calm heart palpitations and irregular heartbeats, making it particularly beneficial for individuals who experience these symptoms due to stress or anxiety. Its mildly sedative effects help to regulate the heart's rhythm.
- **Lowers Blood Pressure:** Motherwort has vasodilating properties, which help to widen blood vessels, improving circulation and reducing blood pressure. This makes it a natural remedy for mild hypertension.
- **Calms the Nervous System:** Motherwort's relaxing properties help to reduce stress and anxiety, both of which can strain the heart. It is often used to relieve heart palpitations linked to emotional stress.
- **Strengthens the Heart:** The compounds in motherwort have been shown to improve the strength and function of the heart muscle, supporting overall cardiovascular health. It is particularly helpful for those with weak heart function or those recovering from heart conditions.
- **Supports Female Reproductive Health:** In addition to its heart-supporting benefits, motherwort is also known for its role in supporting female reproductive health, particularly in easing menstrual cramps and regulating menstrual cycles.

How to Make Motherwort Heart Support Tea:

Ingredients:
- 1 tablespoon dried motherwort leaves (or 2 tablespoons fresh leaves)
- 2 cups water
- Optional: 1 teaspoon honey or a slice of lemon for added flavor

Instructions:

1. Bring the water to a boil in a small saucepan.
2. Add the dried or fresh motherwort leaves to the boiling water.
3. Reduce the heat and let the leaves simmer for 10-15 minutes to extract the beneficial compounds.
4. Remove from heat and let the tea steep for an additional 5 minutes.
5. Strain the tea into a cup, discarding the leaves. Add honey or lemon to taste, if desired.
6. Drink the tea warm, and store any leftover tea in the refrigerator for up to two days.

Dosage:

- For general heart support: Drink 1 cup of motherwort tea daily.
- For anxiety and palpitations: Drink 1-2 cups of tea as needed to help calm the heart and nervous system.

Science Behind Motherwort's Benefits for Heart Health:

Motherwort contains several active compounds, including alkaloids like leonurine, which have been studied for their ability to strengthen the heart muscle and improve circulation. These compounds also have mild sedative properties that help to regulate heart rhythm and reduce palpitations. Research published in the *Journal of Ethnopharmacology* has shown that motherwort has positive effects on blood pressure and heart rate, particularly in individuals with anxiety-induced heart issues. Additionally, motherwort's flavonoid content provides antioxidant protection, helping to prevent oxidative damage to the cardiovascular system.

Variations and Additions:

- **Motherwort and Hawthorn Heart Tea:** Combining motherwort with hawthorn, another heart-healthy herb, can enhance cardiovascular support, particularly for individuals with weak heart function or high blood pressure.
- **Motherwort and Lemon Balm Relaxing Tea:** Adding lemon balm to motherwort tea provides additional calming effects, making it an excellent remedy for stress-related heart palpitations and anxiety.
- **Motherwort and Lavender Heart Tea:** Lavender's soothing properties complement motherwort's heart-supporting benefits, creating a tea that helps relieve tension and promote relaxation.
- **Motherwort and Passionflower Tea:** Passionflower's calming properties enhance motherwort's ability to reduce anxiety and support heart health, particularly in individuals prone to stress.

Additional Benefits of Motherwort:

- **Reduces Menstrual Cramps:** Motherwort is known to help ease menstrual discomfort by relaxing the uterine muscles, making it beneficial for women who experience painful periods.
- **Supports Postpartum Recovery:** Historically, motherwort has been used to help women recover after childbirth by supporting uterine health and reducing postpartum anxiety.
- **Alleviates Anxiety:** Due to its mild sedative properties, motherwort is commonly used to reduce symptoms of anxiety and nervous tension, helping to calm both the heart and mind.
- **Promotes Digestive Health:** Motherwort's relaxing effects on smooth muscles can also help to relieve digestive discomfort, particularly when stress is a contributing factor.

Precautions:

- **Medication Interactions:** Motherwort may interact with certain heart medications, including blood pressure medications and sedatives. Consult a healthcare provider before using motherwort if you are taking any prescription medications.
- **Pregnancy and Breastfeeding:** Motherwort should be avoided during pregnancy, as it may stimulate uterine contractions. Consult a healthcare provider before using motherwort if you are breastfeeding.
- **Allergies and Sensitivities:** Some individuals may experience allergic reactions to motherwort. If you have a known sensitivity to plants in the mint family (Lamiaceae), use motherwort with caution.
- **Low Blood Pressure:** If you have low blood pressure, use motherwort cautiously, as it may further lower your blood pressure.

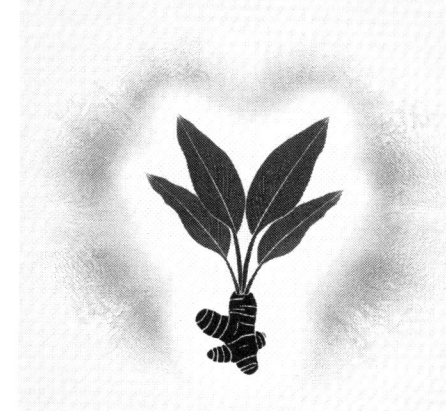

5. Turmeric Anti-Inflammatory Latte

Turmeric Anti-Inflammatory Latte is a warm, soothing beverage made from turmeric, a golden spice renowned for its powerful anti-inflammatory and antioxidant properties. Known in traditional Ayurvedic medicine as a healing tonic, turmeric contains curcumin, its main active compound, which has been extensively studied for its ability to reduce inflammation, improve digestion, and support joint health. This latte, often referred to as "golden milk," is especially beneficial for individuals dealing with chronic inflammation, arthritis, or those seeking a natural way to enhance their overall well-being.

Key Benefits of Turmeric Anti-Inflammatory Latte:

- **Reduces Inflammation:** Turmeric is rich in curcumin, a potent anti-inflammatory compound that helps to reduce chronic inflammation linked to conditions like arthritis, heart disease, and autoimmune disorders. Regular consumption of this latte may help alleviate joint pain and stiffness.
- **Boosts Immune Function:** Turmeric's antioxidant properties help strengthen the immune system by protecting cells from oxidative stress and free radical damage. This makes it an excellent choice for supporting immune health, especially during cold and flu season.
- **Supports Joint Health:** The anti-inflammatory effects of curcumin make this latte particularly beneficial for individuals with joint pain or arthritis. It helps to reduce swelling and improve mobility.
- **Improves Digestion:** Turmeric has been traditionally used to support digestion by stimulating bile production and reducing bloating and gas. The warming spices in this latte, such as ginger or cinnamon, further enhance its digestive benefits.
- **Rich in Antioxidants:** Curcumin, along with other spices like cinnamon and ginger, provides a powerful dose of antioxidants that protect the body from oxidative damage, promoting overall health and longevity.

How to Make Turmeric Anti-Inflammatory Latte:

Ingredients:

- 1 teaspoon ground turmeric
(or 1 tablespoon fresh grated turmeric)
- 1 cup milk
(dairy, almond, coconut, or oat milk)
- ½ teaspoon ground cinnamon
- ½ teaspoon ground ginger
(or 1 teaspoon fresh grated ginger)
- 1 teaspoon honey or maple syrup
(optional, for sweetness)
- Pinch of black pepper
(to enhance curcumin absorption)
- Optional: 1 teaspoon coconut oil or ghee for added richness and health benefits

Instructions:

In a small saucepan, heat the milk over medium heat until warm but not boiling.

1. Add the turmeric, cinnamon, ginger, and black pepper to the warm milk. Stir well to combine.

2. If using coconut oil or ghee, stir it into the mixture for a creamier texture and additional health benefits.

3. Simmer the mixture for 5-10 minutes, allowing the spices to infuse into the milk. Stir occasionally to prevent the spices from settling at the bottom.

4. Remove from heat and let it cool slightly. Strain the mixture into a mug to remove any spice residue.

5. Stir in honey or maple syrup to taste, and enjoy your warm, soothing turmeric latte.

Dosage:

- For general anti-inflammatory support: Enjoy 1 cup of turmeric latte daily, especially in the evening for its calming effects.
- For joint pain or arthritis: Drink 1-2 cups daily to help reduce inflammation and support joint mobility.

Science Behind Turmeric's Benefits for Inflammation:

Turmeric's primary active compound, curcumin, has been extensively researched for its anti-inflammatory and antioxidant properties. Curcumin works by inhibiting molecules like NF-κB, which play a significant role in chronic inflammation. Studies published in *Phytotherapy Research* and *The Journal of Alternative and Complementary Medicine* highlight turmeric's effectiveness in reducing joint pain and stiffness in individuals with arthritis, as well as its role in preventing inflammatory diseases. Black pepper, added to the latte, contains piperine, which significantly enhances the absorption of curcumin in the body, making this combination more effective.

Variations and Additions:

- **Turmeric and Ginger Latte:** For an extra anti-inflammatory boost, increase the amount of ginger, which has its own powerful anti-inflammatory properties and supports digestion.
- **Turmeric and Ashwagandha Latte:** Ashwagandha is an adaptogen that helps the body manage stress and reduce cortisol levels. Adding ashwagandha to your latte can enhance relaxation and reduce inflammation.
- **Turmeric and Cinnamon Latte:** Cinnamon adds additional antioxidants and helps regulate blood sugar levels, making this a perfect blend for those with metabolic concerns.
- **Turmeric and Matcha Latte:** For an energizing twist, add a teaspoon of matcha powder. Matcha provides a gentle caffeine boost along with its own antioxidant properties, complementing the anti-inflammatory effects of turmeric.

Additional Benefits of Turmeric Anti-Inflammatory Latte:

- **Promotes Relaxation and Sleep:** Drinking a turmeric latte in the evening can help relax the body and mind, as its warming spices promote a sense of calm. This makes it a wonderful bedtime beverage.
- **Supports Liver Health:** Turmeric has been shown to enhance liver detoxification processes, helping to cleanse the body of toxins and support overall liver function.
- **Enhances Skin Health:** The antioxidants in turmeric and other spices can help improve skin health by reducing inflammation, fighting free radicals, and promoting a healthy glow.
- **Aids in Weight Management:** Turmeric may help support metabolism and reduce inflammation associated with obesity, making it a useful tool for those looking to manage their weight naturally.

Precautions:

- **Medication Interactions:** Turmeric may interact with certain medications, including blood thinners and medications for diabetes. Consult your healthcare provider before consuming turmeric in medicinal doses if you are on these medications.
- **Pregnancy and Breastfeeding:** While turmeric is generally safe in culinary amounts, high doses of turmeric should be avoided during pregnancy, as it may stimulate uterine contractions. Consult a healthcare provider before using turmeric supplements if you are breastfeeding.
- **Gastrointestinal Sensitivity:** Some individuals may experience gastrointestinal discomfort, such as bloating or acid reflux, when consuming large amounts of turmeric. Start with small amounts and gradually increase the dosage as needed.

Chapter 7

Nurturing Skin Health

- Common Skin Conditions and Natural Solutions
- Top 5 Herbal Recipes for Radiant Skin
  1. Aloe Vera Healing Gel
  2. Calendula Skin Salve
  3. Tea Tree Acne Spot Treatment
  4. Rose Water Facial Toner
  5. Oatmeal and Honey Exfoliant

Common Skin Conditions and Natural Solutions

Common Skin Conditions and Natural Solutions provides an effective, holistic approach to managing everyday skin issues by using natural remedies that soothe, heal, and support the skin's health. Just as garlic and olive oil work synergistically to promote cardiovascular health, many natural ingredients offer profound benefits for common skin conditions. These conditions, from dryness and irritation to more chronic issues like eczema or acne, can often be improved by tapping into nature's inherent healing power.

Key Benefits of Natural Solutions for Common Skin Conditions:

- **Reduces Inflammation**: Natural ingredients like **aloe vera**, **turmeric**, and **chamomile** contain anti-inflammatory properties that calm redness and swelling, helping to reduce the discomfort associated with conditions like eczema, psoriasis, or acne.

- **Promotes Hydration**: Ingredients such as **coconut oil** and **shea butter** help lock in moisture, supporting the skin's barrier function and preventing dryness or flaking, essential for those with sensitive or dry skin types.

- **Soothes Irritation**: Many skin conditions involve itching or irritation. **Colloidal oatmeal** and **calendula** are known for their soothing effects, providing relief from conditions like contact dermatitis or allergic reactions.

- **Supports Skin Healing**: **Honey**, with its antimicrobial and wound-healing properties, and **aloe vera**, known for its ability to speed up skin regeneration, can help the skin heal faster, reducing scarring and irritation.

- **Balances Oil Production**: Natural ingredients such as **tea tree oil** and **witch hazel** are effective in managing oily skin and acne by reducing excess sebum production without stripping the skin of its natural oils.

Common Skin Conditions and Natural Solutions:

1. **Eczema**:

    - **Symptoms**: Dry, itchy, and inflamed skin, often on the hands, face, or behind the knees.
    - **Natural Solution**: Apply **coconut oil** or **shea butter** daily to moisturize the skin. Taking an **oatmeal bath** soothes itching and reduces inflammation. **Aloe vera gel** helps calm flare-ups.

2. **Acne**:

    - **Symptoms**: Clogged pores leading to pimples, blackheads, and whiteheads, commonly on the face, chest, and back.
    - **Natural Solution**: Use **tea tree oil** diluted with a carrier oil to kill acne-causing bacteria. **Honey and cinnamon masks** help fight inflammation, while **witch hazel** acts as a natural toner to balance oil levels.

Ch. 7 - Nurturing Skin Health

3. **Psoriasis**:

   - **Symptoms**: Red, scaly patches of skin, often covered with a silvery sheen, typically on the scalp, knees, or elbows.
   - **Natural Solution**: **Aloe vera gel** soothes and hydrates dry patches. **Turmeric paste** can reduce inflammation and flare-ups, while soaking in a **Dead Sea salt bath** helps to remove dead skin.

4. **Rosacea**:

   - **Symptoms**: Facial redness, visible blood vessels, and small, red bumps on the cheeks and nose.
   - **Natural Solution**: Use a **green tea compress** to reduce redness and inflammation. **Chamomile tea** applied as a wash soothes irritated skin, and **aloe vera gel** calms flare-ups.

5. **Contact Dermatitis**:

   - **Symptoms**: Red, itchy, and sometimes blistered skin caused by contact with an irritant or allergen.
   - **Natural Solution**: Apply **calendula ointment** to reduce swelling and itching. **Apple cider vinegar** diluted in water helps restore the skin's pH balance. **Oatmeal paste** soothes and relieves itching.

6. **Fungal Infections**:

   - **Symptoms**: Red, itchy patches of skin, often affecting the feet (athlete's foot) or body (ringworm).
   - **Natural Solution**: Use **tea tree oil** for its antifungal properties, applying it to affected areas twice daily. **Garlic** paste or supplements can also fight fungal infections. **Coconut oil** helps soothe the skin and reduce fungal growth.

7. **Hyperpigmentation**:

   - **Symptoms**: Dark spots or patches on the skin, often caused by sun exposure or acne scars.
   - **Natural Solution**: Apply **licorice extract** or **vitamin C serum** to lighten dark spots over time. **Aloe vera gel** can help reduce pigmentation and even out skin tone.

8. **Dandruff**:

   - **Symptoms**: Flaky, itchy scalp caused by dryness or a yeast overgrowth.
   - **Natural Solution**: Rinse the scalp with **apple cider vinegar** to balance pH and reduce yeast growth. **Tea tree oil** added to shampoo helps reduce flakes, and **aloe vera** soothes scalp irritation.

Science Behind Natural Ingredients for Skin Health:

Natural ingredients like **aloe vera**, **coconut oil**, and **tea tree oil** are rich in compounds that provide protective, soothing, and healing benefits. **Aloe vera** contains **polysaccharides**, which speed up skin healing, while **coconut oil** is packed with **fatty acids** that maintain the skin's barrier and hydrate deeply. Studies published in *Dermatology Research and Practice* highlight the antimicrobial effects of **tea tree oil**, which is effective against acne-causing bacteria.

Herbs such as **calendula** and **chamomile** are rich in **flavonoids** and **triterpenoids**, which have anti-inflammatory and soothing effects on irritated skin, making them ideal for treating dermatitis or rosacea. Scientific studies on **licorice extract**, published in the *Journal of Drugs in Dermatology*, show its ability to reduce hyperpigmentation by inhibiting melanin production, promoting a more even skin tone.

Variations and Additions:

- **Herbal Infused Oil**: Infuse oils like olive or almond with herbs such as **calendula** or **lavender** to enhance their soothing and anti-inflammatory properties. These can be used for eczema, psoriasis, or dermatitis.

- **Aloe Vera and Honey Gel**: Combine **aloe vera** with **honey** for added moisture and healing. Honey's antibacterial properties, combined with aloe's cooling effects, make it ideal for acne or minor burns.

- **Turmeric and Coconut Oil Mask**: A mix of **turmeric** and **coconut oil** can be applied to reduce the appearance of acne scars and brighten dull skin.

- **Green Tea Ice Cubes**: Freeze **green tea** into ice cubes and rub them over inflamed skin or acne-prone areas for an instant calming effect.

Additional Benefits of Natural Ingredients:

- **Anti-Aging**: Ingredients like **vitamin C** and **green tea** are rich in antioxidants that help combat free radicals, reducing the appearance of wrinkles and fine lines.

- **Reduces Redness**: **Licorice extract** and **aloe vera** help calm red, inflamed skin, making them useful for conditions like rosacea and acne.

- **Moisturizes Dry Skin**: **Coconut oil** and **shea butter** deeply hydrate and repair dry, cracked skin, ideal for eczema or psoriasis sufferers.

- **Protects Against Environmental Stress**: **Green tea** and **turmeric** contain antioxidants that protect the skin from UV rays and pollution.

Precautions:

- **Allergic Reactions**: Some individuals may have allergies to natural ingredients such as **tea tree oil**, **coconut oil**, or **calendula**. Always perform a patch test before using any new remedy.

- **Photosensitivity**: Ingredients like **citrus essential oils** (found in lemon or lime) can cause the skin to become more sensitive to the sun. Avoid direct sunlight after using products containing these oils.

- **Medical Conditions**: For individuals with severe skin conditions such as psoriasis or eczema, it's important to consult a healthcare provider before using natural remedies in conjunction with prescribed treatments.

Top 5 Herbal Recipes for Radiant Skin

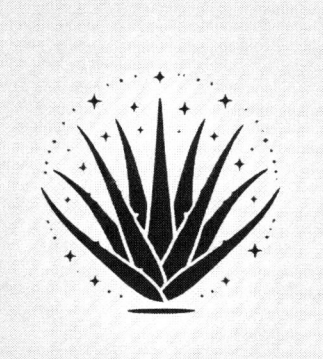

1. Aloe Vera Healing Gel

Aloe Vera Healing Gel is a soothing and restorative natural remedy made from the inner gel of the *Aloe barbadensis* plant, commonly known as aloe vera. This gel has been used for centuries to treat a variety of skin conditions due to its hydrating, anti-inflammatory, and healing properties. Aloe vera is packed with vitamins, minerals, enzymes, and antioxidants that help soothe irritation, accelerate wound healing, and nourish the skin. Whether applied to burns, cuts, or dry skin, aloe vera healing gel is a versatile solution for promoting overall skin health.

Key Benefits of Aloe Vera Healing Gel:

- **Soothes Burns and Sunburns**: Aloe vera's cooling and hydrating properties make it highly effective for treating minor burns and sunburns. Its high water content helps replenish moisture in damaged skin, while its anti-inflammatory properties reduce redness and swelling.
- **Accelerates Wound Healing**: Aloe vera contains polysaccharides and gibberellins, which promote cell regeneration and help the skin heal faster. It is particularly beneficial for minor cuts, scrapes, and wounds.
- **Reduces Inflammation**: Aloe's rich content of **beta-sitosterol** and **salicylic acid** provides anti-inflammatory benefits, making it an effective remedy for irritated or inflamed skin caused by conditions like eczema, psoriasis, or acne.
- **Hydrates and Moisturizes**: Aloe vera is composed of 99% water and provides deep hydration without leaving a greasy residue. It penetrates the skin easily, making it a great natural moisturizer for dry or dehydrated skin.
- **Rich in Antioxidants**: Aloe vera contains vitamins **A**, **C**, and **E**, which are antioxidants that help protect the skin from environmental damage and promote the healing of damaged tissues.

How to Make Aloe Vera Healing Gel:

Ingredients:

- 1 large aloe vera leaf (or store-bought pure aloe vera gel)
- 1 teaspoon vitamin E oil (optional, for added skin nourishment)
- 2-3 drops essential oil (optional, for fragrance and added skin benefits; lavender or tea tree oil are excellent choices)

Instructions:

1. If using a fresh aloe vera leaf, cut it open lengthwise and scoop out the clear gel from the inside of the leaf using a spoon.
2. Place the gel in a blender and blend it for a few seconds until it becomes smooth and slightly frothy.
3. Optional: Add vitamin E oil for extra nourishment and a few drops of essential oil if you prefer a scented gel or additional benefits like lavender for soothing or tea tree for acne-prone skin.
4. Pour the aloe vera gel into a clean, airtight jar or container. It can be stored in the refrigerator for up to a week to maintain its freshness and potency.

How to Use:

- **For Burns or Sunburn**: Apply the aloe vera healing gel directly to the affected area. Its cooling and hydrating properties will immediately help soothe the burn. Reapply as needed throughout the day.

Ch. 7 - Top 5 Herbal Recipes for Radiant Skin

- **For Cuts or Wounds**: Gently cleanse the wound and apply a small amount of the gel to promote faster healing and protect the skin from infection.
- **For Dry Skin**: Use the gel as a daily moisturizer on the face or body. It absorbs quickly and leaves the skin feeling soft and hydrated without clogging pores.
- **For Acne**: Apply a thin layer of aloe vera gel to acne-prone areas to reduce inflammation and redness. Its antibacterial properties help keep the skin clear and reduce the frequency of breakouts.

Science Behind Aloe Vera's Healing Properties:

Aloe vera's healing power is rooted in its rich composition of **polysaccharides**, which help retain moisture and support skin repair, and **glycoproteins**, which reduce inflammation and pain. Research published in *Skin Pharmacology and Physiology* highlights aloe vera's ability to accelerate wound healing by promoting collagen production and increasing the tensile strength of healing skin. Aloe vera's high water content and **salicylic acid** also help calm inflammation, making it ideal for treating burns, acne, and other skin irritations.

The plant's antioxidant profile, including vitamins A, C, and E, protects the skin from free radical damage, which is a key factor in slowing down the aging process. Aloe's antimicrobial properties, especially in fighting bacteria like *Staphylococcus* and *Pseudomonas*, make it a reliable choice for treating minor wounds and preventing infection.

Variations and Additions:

- **Aloe Vera and Honey Healing Gel**: Mix a teaspoon of honey with aloe vera gel for additional moisture and antimicrobial benefits. Honey also aids in wound healing and soothes irritated skin.
- **Aloe Vera and Coconut Oil Gel**: For an extra hydration boost, mix a small amount of melted coconut oil with the aloe vera gel. This combination is especially effective for very dry or rough skin.
- **Aloe Vera and Cucumber Gel**: Blend cucumber juice with aloe vera gel for a refreshing and hydrating remedy. Cucumber adds extra cooling effects, making it ideal for sunburns and skin inflammation.
- **Aloe Vera and Turmeric Gel**: Add a pinch of turmeric powder for its anti-inflammatory and brightening properties. This blend can help reduce redness and hyperpigmentation.

Additional Benefits of Aloe Vera Healing Gel:

- **Anti-Aging Properties**: Aloe vera stimulates the production of collagen and elastin, improving skin elasticity and reducing the appearance of fine lines and wrinkles.
- **Reduces Hyperpigmentation**: Regular use of aloe vera can help lighten dark spots and improve skin tone by promoting the natural regeneration of skin cells.
- **Soothes Razor Burn**: Aloe vera's cooling and anti-inflammatory effects help reduce irritation and redness caused by shaving.
- **Protects Against Environmental Damage**: Aloe's antioxidant content protects the skin from environmental stressors such as pollution and UV damage, reducing the risk of premature aging.

Precautions:

- **Allergic Reactions**: While aloe vera is generally safe for most people, some may experience allergic reactions such as redness, itching, or swelling. It's best to perform a patch test on a small area of skin before widespread use.
- **Storage**: Store homemade aloe vera gel in the refrigerator to extend its shelf life. Fresh gel can last up to one week, while store-bought aloe vera gel often contains preservatives and can last longer.
- **Latex Sensitivity**: The outer layer of the aloe plant contains a substance called **aloe latex**, which can be irritating. Ensure only the inner gel is used when preparing homemade aloe vera products.

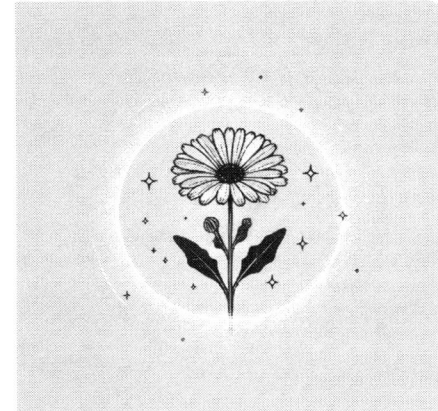

2. Calendula Skin Salve

Calendula Skin Salve is a soothing and healing natural remedy made from the flowers of the *Calendula officinalis* plant, also known as marigold. Calendula has long been valued for its anti-inflammatory, antimicrobial, and skin-repairing properties, making it ideal for treating a variety of skin conditions, including dry skin, cuts, scrapes, burns, and rashes. This skin salve combines the healing power of calendula with nourishing oils and beeswax, creating a protective balm that can be applied to irritated or damaged skin, helping to accelerate healing and soothe discomfort.

Key Benefits of Calendula Skin Salve:

- **Promotes Wound Healing**: Calendula is known for its ability to speed up the healing process of minor wounds, cuts, and abrasions by stimulating collagen production and tissue regeneration. It also helps reduce the risk of infection.
- **Reduces Inflammation**: The anti-inflammatory compounds in calendula, such as flavonoids and triterpenoids, help calm irritated or inflamed skin, making this salve ideal for conditions like eczema, dermatitis, or diaper rash.
- **Moisturizes Dry, Cracked Skin**: Calendula salve provides deep hydration and helps restore the skin's natural moisture barrier, making it beneficial for dry, cracked, or rough skin, especially on hands, feet, and elbows.
- **Soothes Burns and Sunburns**: Calendula's cooling and anti-inflammatory properties help reduce redness, pain, and swelling associated with burns or sunburns. It promotes faster recovery by moisturizing and calming damaged skin.
- **Antimicrobial Properties**: Calendula has mild antimicrobial effects, which help prevent infections in cuts, scrapes, and minor burns. This makes it particularly useful for skin that's vulnerable to bacterial growth.

How to Make Calendula Skin Salve:

Ingredients:
- 1 cup dried calendula flowers
- 1 cup carrier oil (such as olive oil, coconut oil, or almond oil)
- 1/4 cup beeswax (for thickening the salve)
- Optional: 1 teaspoon vitamin E oil (for added nourishment and preservation)
- Optional: A few drops of lavender or tea tree essential oil (for additional soothing and antimicrobial benefits)

Instructions:

1. Infuse the Calendula Oil: In a double boiler, gently heat the dried calendula flowers with your chosen carrier oil. Simmer on low heat for 2-3 hours, allowing the calendula to infuse its healing properties into the oil. Stir occasionally to ensure the flowers are well-soaked in the oil.

2. Strain the Oil: After the infusion is complete, strain the oil through a fine mesh strainer or cheesecloth, pressing the flowers to extract as much of the oil as possible. Discard the flowers and set the calendula-infused oil aside.

3. Melt the Beeswax: In a clean double boiler, melt the beeswax over low heat. Once fully melted, slowly add the calendula-infused oil, stirring continuously to combine the two ingredients.

4. Add Extras: If using, stir in the vitamin E oil and essential oils (lavender for calming or tea tree for antimicrobial benefits). Mix well to combine all the ingredients.

5. Pour and Cool: Pour the mixture into small glass jars or tins. Allow the salve to cool and solidify at room temperature. Once cooled, cover the containers with lids and store in a cool, dry place.

How to Use:

- **For Minor Cuts and Scrapes**: Clean the affected area and apply a small amount of calendula salve to promote healing and prevent infection.
- **For Dry or Cracked Skin**: Massage the salve into dry or cracked skin, especially on areas like the hands, feet, and elbows, to restore moisture and prevent further irritation.
- **For Burns and Sunburns**: Gently apply the salve to the affected areas to reduce redness, pain, and inflammation, and to speed up the skin's recovery process.
- **For Diaper Rash**: Use calendula salve on babies to soothe diaper rash and protect sensitive skin from further irritation.

Science Behind Calendula's Healing Properties:

Calendula contains active compounds like **flavonoids**, **triterpenoids**, and **carotenoids**, which give it powerful anti-inflammatory, antioxidant, and healing properties. These compounds work to reduce inflammation, stimulate tissue regeneration, and protect the skin from oxidative stress. Research published in the *Journal of Wound Care* has shown that calendula can significantly speed up the healing process of wounds by increasing collagen production and enhancing tissue repair.

Calendula's **antimicrobial** properties help prevent infections, making it particularly useful for treating minor cuts, burns, and scrapes. Its ability to inhibit the growth of bacteria like *Staphylococcus aureus* and *Candida albicans* reduces the likelihood of infections, while its antioxidant properties protect the skin from environmental damage and premature aging.

Variations and Additions:

- **Calendula and Chamomile Skin Salve**: Add dried chamomile flowers to the calendula oil infusion for extra soothing benefits. Chamomile is known for its calming effects on irritated and sensitive skin.
- **Calendula and Lavender Salve**: Incorporate lavender essential oil for additional anti-inflammatory and calming properties. This is especially helpful for stress-related skin conditions like eczema or dermatitis.
- **Calendula and Arnica Salve**: Add arnica oil to the mixture for a salve that helps reduce bruising and muscle soreness, making it ideal for athletes or those with minor injuries.
- **Calendula and Coconut Oil Salve**: Use coconut oil as the carrier oil for its added antibacterial and moisturizing benefits, enhancing the healing properties of the salve.

Additional Benefits of Calendula Skin Salve:

- **Helps with Eczema and Dermatitis**: Calendula's anti-inflammatory and moisturizing properties provide relief from the itchiness and irritation caused by eczema and dermatitis.
- **Reduces Scarring**: Calendula's ability to promote collagen production can help reduce the appearance of scars, stretch marks, and other skin imperfections.
- **Gentle for Sensitive Skin**: Calendula is known for being gentle enough for even the most sensitive skin types, making it a great choice for babies or people with allergies.
- **Soothes Insect Bites and Stings**: Calendula's anti-inflammatory and cooling effects can relieve the itching and discomfort caused by insect bites, bee stings, and other skin irritations.

Precautions:

- **Allergies**: While calendula is generally safe for most people, those with allergies to plants in the **Asteraceae** family (such as daisies, marigolds, or ragweed) may experience an allergic reaction. Always perform a patch test before applying calendula salve to a large area of skin.
- **Storage**: Keep the calendula salve in a cool, dry place, and it will last for up to a year. If stored in a refrigerator, its shelf life can be extended further.
- **Avoid Ingestion**: Calendula salve is intended for external use only. Avoid using it on deep wounds or serious burns unless directed by a healthcare provider.

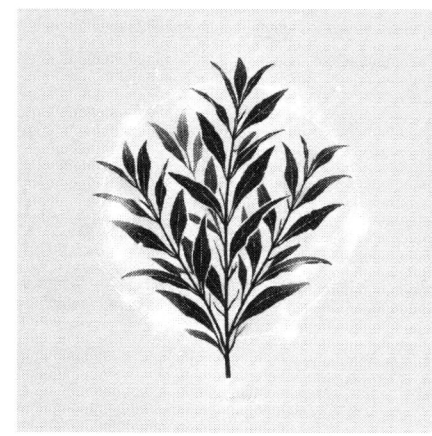

3. Tea Tree Acne Spot Treatment

Tea Tree Acne Spot Treatment is a powerful natural remedy that utilizes the antibacterial and anti-inflammatory properties of tea tree oil to target and reduce acne. Tea tree oil, derived from the leaves of the *Melaleuca alternifolia* plant, has been used for centuries to treat skin infections and inflammation. This spot treatment is particularly effective for reducing pimples, redness, and swelling without the harsh side effects of synthetic acne treatments. It works by killing acne-causing bacteria, soothing irritated skin, and promoting faster healing of blemishes.

Key Benefits of Tea Tree Acne Spot Treatment:

- **Fights Acne-Causing Bacteria**: Tea tree oil contains **terpinen-4-ol**, which is known for its strong antibacterial properties. It penetrates the skin to kill *Propionibacterium acnes*, the bacteria responsible for causing acne, reducing the size and severity of breakouts.
- **Reduces Redness and Swelling**: Tea tree oil's anti-inflammatory properties help calm inflamed skin, reducing redness and swelling around pimples, making them less noticeable and less painful.
- **Promotes Healing**: Tea tree oil helps speed up the healing process of acne lesions by drying out the blemish and preventing the formation of new breakouts. Its antiseptic properties also reduce the risk of scarring and further infection.
- **Gentle on Skin**: Unlike some chemical-based acne treatments that can cause dryness and irritation, tea tree oil is gentler on the skin and can be used on sensitive areas when diluted properly.
- **Balances Oil Production**: Tea tree oil can help regulate the skin's oil production, making it especially beneficial for those with oily or combination skin. By preventing excess oil buildup, it reduces the likelihood of future breakouts.

How to Make Tea Tree Acne Spot Treatment:

Ingredients:
- 1 teaspoon carrier oil (such as jojoba oil, almond oil, or grapeseed oil)
- 1-2 drops of 100% pure tea tree essential oil
- Optional: 1 drop of lavender essential oil (for additional soothing and anti-inflammatory effects)

Instructions:

1. In a small bowl or container, mix 1-2 drops of tea tree oil with 1 teaspoon of your chosen carrier oil. Tea tree oil is potent and should be diluted with a carrier oil to prevent skin irritation.
2. Optional: Add a drop of lavender essential oil to the mixture for its calming and skin-soothing properties.
3. Stir the mixture well to combine the oils.

How to Use:

- **Spot Treatment for Pimples**: Using a clean cotton swab or your fingertip, apply the tea tree oil mixture directly to individual pimples or affected areas. Avoid applying the mixture to large areas of the skin, as tea tree oil is strong and meant for targeted treatment.

- **Leave on Overnight**: For best results, leave the treatment on overnight to allow the tea tree oil to penetrate the skin and work on the blemish. In the morning, cleanse your face as usual.
- **Use 1-2 Times Daily**: Repeat the application once or twice daily as needed, especially during active breakouts, until the pimple subsides.

Science Behind Tea Tree Oil's Acne-Fighting Properties:

Tea tree oil's active ingredient, **terpinen-4-ol**, has been studied for its potent antimicrobial and anti-inflammatory properties. According to research published in the *Journal of Dermatology*, tea tree oil has been shown to effectively reduce both the number of acne lesions and the severity of acne symptoms when used regularly. Its ability to kill *Propionibacterium acnes* bacteria and reduce inflammation makes it a natural alternative to conventional acne treatments, such as benzoyl peroxide, with fewer side effects like dryness and irritation.

Tea tree oil's natural antiseptic properties also help prevent the formation of new acne lesions by keeping pores clear of bacteria and debris. Studies have shown that tea tree oil can reduce acne by up to 40-50% over several weeks when used consistently.

Variations and Additions:

- **Tea Tree and Aloe Vera Spot Treatment**: Mix a few drops of tea tree oil with pure aloe vera gel for a cooling and hydrating spot treatment. Aloe vera helps reduce inflammation and redness, while also keeping the skin moisturized.
- **Tea Tree and Witch Hazel Toner**: Combine tea tree oil with witch hazel to create an acne-fighting toner. Witch hazel helps tighten pores and reduce oil production, making it a great combination with tea tree oil.
- **Tea Tree and Honey Spot Treatment**: Honey has natural antibacterial and anti-inflammatory properties that complement tea tree oil. Mix a small amount of honey with tea tree oil and apply it as a spot treatment for more hydration and soothing.

Additional Benefits of Tea Tree Acne Spot Treatment:

- **Reduces Blackheads and Whiteheads**: Tea tree oil's ability to regulate oil production helps prevent clogged pores, reducing the formation of blackheads and whiteheads.
- **Prevents Future Breakouts**: Regular use of tea tree oil as part of a skincare routine can help prevent the recurrence of acne by keeping the skin clear of bacteria and excess oil.
- **Gentle for Sensitive Skin**: When properly diluted, tea tree oil is safe for sensitive skin and can be used on areas prone to irritation, such as the face and neck.
- **Soothes Razor Burn**: Tea tree oil can also be used to soothe razor burn or ingrown hairs, reducing redness and irritation after shaving.

Precautions:

- **Dilution is Key**: Pure tea tree oil is potent and should always be diluted with a carrier oil before applying it to the skin. Undiluted tea tree oil can cause irritation, dryness, or even an allergic reaction in some individuals.
- **Patch Test First**: Before applying tea tree oil to your face, perform a patch test on a small area of skin (such as the inside of your wrist) to check for any allergic reactions or sensitivity.
- **Avoid Eye Area**: Tea tree oil should not be applied near the eyes, as it can cause irritation. If contact occurs, rinse thoroughly with water.
- **Storage**: Store tea tree oil in a cool, dark place to preserve its potency. Essential oils can degrade when exposed to light or heat.

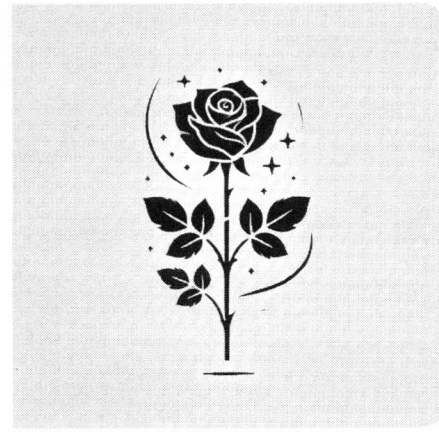

4. Rose Water Facial Toner

Rose Water Facial Toner is a refreshing and gentle skincare remedy made from distilled rose petals. Known for its soothing and hydrating properties, rose water is an excellent natural toner that helps balance the skin's pH, reduce redness, and tighten pores. Rose water is suitable for all skin types, particularly sensitive and dry skin, and can be used as part of a daily skincare routine to refresh the face, improve complexion, and promote a healthy glow. This toner is not only rejuvenating but also filled with antioxidants that protect and nourish the skin.

Key Benefits of Rose Water Facial Toner:

- **Balances Skin's pH**: Rose water helps to naturally balance the skin's pH levels, which can be disrupted by harsh cleansers or environmental factors. By restoring balance, it helps prevent excess oil production and dryness.
- **Soothes Irritation and Reduces Redness**: Rose water has anti-inflammatory properties that soothe irritated skin, making it ideal for conditions like acne, rosacea, or eczema. It helps calm redness and reduce swelling, promoting a more even skin tone.
- **Hydrates and Refreshes**: With its high water content, rose water provides lightweight hydration to the skin, making it feel refreshed and revitalized. It can also help prep the skin for better absorption of moisturizers or serums.
- **Tightens Pores**: Rose water acts as a natural astringent, tightening pores and helping to prevent dirt and impurities from clogging them. This helps keep the skin smooth and reduces the appearance of large pores.
- **Rich in Antioxidants**: Packed with vitamins **A**, **C**, and **E**, rose water provides antioxidant protection that helps combat free radical damage, keeping the skin youthful and radiant.

How to Make Rose Water Facial Toner:

Ingredients:
- 1/2 cup pure rose water
(can be store-bought or homemade)
- 1 teaspoon witch hazel
(optional, for additional astringent properties)
- 1 teaspoon aloe vera gel
(optional, for added hydration and soothing)
- 2-3 drops of essential oil (optional, such as lavender or chamomile for extra calming effects)

Instructions:

1. If making rose water at home, gently simmer fresh rose petals in distilled water for 30 minutes, then strain the liquid into a clean jar. Allow it to cool before using.

2. Combine 1/2 cup of pure rose water with 1 teaspoon of witch hazel and 1 teaspoon of aloe vera gel (if using) in a small bottle or spray bottle.

3. Add a few drops of essential oil if desired. Essential oils like lavender or chamomile enhance the calming and soothing effects of the toner.

4. Shake the bottle gently to mix the ingredients. Your rose water toner is now ready to use.

How to Use:

- **As a Daily Toner**: After cleansing your face, apply the rose water toner using a cotton pad or spritz directly onto your skin. Gently pat it into your skin with clean hands, or allow it to air dry before applying moisturizer.
- **Throughout the Day**: Use it as a refreshing facial mist during the day to keep your skin hydrated and calm, especially in dry environments or after exposure to the sun.
- **To Set Makeup**: Lightly spritz rose water over your face after applying makeup to set it and give your skin a dewy, natural glow.

Science Behind Rose Water's Benefits for Skin:

Rose water's **anti-inflammatory** and **antioxidant** properties stem from its rich content of vitamins and compounds like **flavonoids** and **tannins**. These components help calm skin irritation and protect the skin from environmental damage caused by free radicals. Studies have shown that rose water's antibacterial properties can help reduce acne by preventing bacterial growth on the skin's surface.

Additionally, rose water's ability to hydrate the skin makes it a valuable remedy for dryness. It supports the skin's natural barrier by providing lightweight moisture, which is essential for maintaining smooth, supple skin. Its natural **astringent** properties help tighten pores and firm the skin, which reduces the visibility of enlarged pores and keeps the skin looking youthful.

Variations and Additions:

- **Rose Water and Green Tea Toner**: Mix rose water with cooled green tea for an extra boost of antioxidants. Green tea helps fight acne, reduces inflammation, and provides a refreshing sensation.
- **Rose Water and Glycerin Toner**: Add a few drops of glycerin to the rose water for enhanced moisture retention. Glycerin acts as a humectant, drawing moisture into the skin and locking it in.
- **Rose Water and Cucumber Toner**: Blend cucumber juice with rose water for a cooling, hydrating toner that's perfect for reducing puffiness and soothing irritated skin.
- **Rose Water and Witch Hazel Toner**: Combine rose water with witch hazel for extra pore-tightening effects. Witch hazel's natural astringent properties help reduce oil production and keep the skin clear.

Additional Benefits of Rose Water Facial Toner:

- **Reduces Signs of Aging**: Regular use of rose water helps prevent the appearance of fine lines and wrinkles by keeping the skin hydrated and protected from oxidative stress.
- **Controls Excess Oil**: While rose water is hydrating, it also helps regulate oil production, making it ideal for oily or combination skin. It refreshes the skin without clogging pores or causing excess shine.
- **Brightens Skin**: Rose water helps improve skin tone by reducing redness and soothing irritation, leading to a brighter and more even complexion.
- **Prevents Acne Breakouts**: Rose water's antibacterial and astringent properties help reduce acne-causing bacteria on the skin while keeping pores clean and unclogged.

Precautions:

- **Allergies**: While rose water is gentle, some individuals may have sensitivities or allergies to roses or rose water. Always perform a patch test before using it on your face, especially if you have sensitive skin.
- **Storage**: Store rose water toner in a cool, dry place. If you've made homemade rose water, it's best to store it in the refrigerator to maintain freshness and extend its shelf life. Use within two weeks if it's homemade, and within a month if store-bought.
- **Avoid Eye Contact**: While rose water is safe for the skin, it should not be applied directly into the eyes. If contact occurs, rinse thoroughly with water.

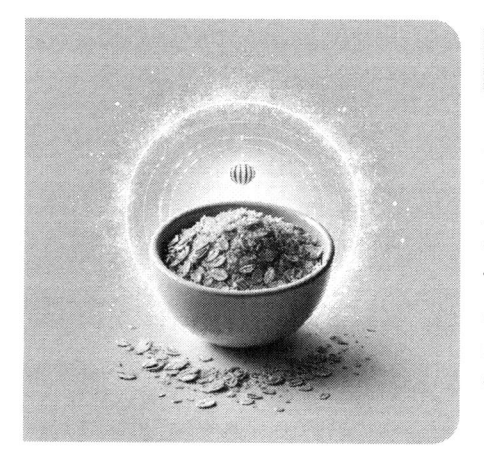

5. Oatmeal and Honey Exfoliant

Oatmeal and Honey Exfoliant is a gentle, natural remedy designed to exfoliate and rejuvenate the skin. Oatmeal is known for its soothing and anti-inflammatory properties, while honey provides deep hydration and acts as a natural humectant, locking moisture into the skin. Together, these ingredients create a mild exfoliant that helps remove dead skin cells, unclog pores, and leave the skin smooth, soft, and radiant. This exfoliant is ideal for all skin types, particularly sensitive or dry skin, as it offers exfoliation without irritation.

Key Benefits of Oatmeal and Honey Exfoliant:

- **Gently Exfoliates**: The finely ground oats in this exfoliant provide a mild physical exfoliation that removes dead skin cells without causing irritation or damage. This helps improve skin texture and reveal a smoother, more radiant complexion.
- **Soothes Irritated Skin**: Oatmeal contains anti-inflammatory compounds such as **avenanthramides**, which help calm redness, itching, and irritation. This makes it ideal for sensitive or irritated skin, especially for those with conditions like eczema or rosacea.
- **Hydrates and Moisturizes**: Honey is a natural humectant, meaning it draws moisture into the skin and helps keep it hydrated. This makes the exfoliant not only effective for removing dead skin cells but also for providing long-lasting moisture.
- **Antibacterial Properties**: Honey has natural antibacterial properties, making it effective in preventing and treating mild acne. It helps keep pores clean and reduces the likelihood of future breakouts.
- **Balances Oil Production**: Both oatmeal and honey help balance the skin's oil production. Oatmeal absorbs excess oil while maintaining the skin's natural moisture, making this exfoliant perfect for both dry and oily skin types.

How to Make Oatmeal and Honey Exfoliant:

Ingredients:
- 2 tablespoons ground oats (finely ground, using a blender or food processor)
- 1 tablespoon raw honey
- 1 teaspoon water or milk §(optional, to thin the mixture if needed)
- Optional: 1 teaspoon yogurt (for added exfoliation and skin-softening benefits)

Instructions:

- In a small bowl, mix 2 tablespoons of finely ground oats with 1 tablespoon of raw honey. Stir until the mixture forms a paste.
- If the mixture is too thick, add 1 teaspoon of water or milk to thin it out. For added benefits, you can mix in a teaspoon of yogurt, which contains lactic acid that gently exfoliates the skin.
- Once combined, your exfoliant is ready to use.

How to Use:

- **For Face**: After cleansing your face, apply the oatmeal and honey mixture in gentle, circular motions, focusing on areas prone to dryness or rough patches. Avoid the delicate eye area.

Let the mixture sit on the skin for 5-10 minutes as a mask, allowing the nutrients to penetrate the skin, then rinse off with warm water.

- **For Body**: This exfoliant can also be used on the body to smooth rough areas like elbows, knees, or the back. Apply in the shower using gentle circular motions, then rinse off thoroughly.

Science Behind Oatmeal and Honey's Benefits for Skin:

Oatmeal is rich in **saponins**, natural compounds that cleanse the skin by removing dirt and oil without stripping away its natural moisture. The **beta-glucan** in oats helps form a protective barrier on the skin, locking in moisture and providing relief from dry or itchy skin. Studies published in the *Journal of Drugs in Dermatology* have demonstrated oatmeal's effectiveness in treating conditions like eczema, where soothing and hydrating properties are essential.

Honey, particularly raw honey, is packed with enzymes, antioxidants, and antibacterial compounds like **methylglyoxal**, which help fight acne-causing bacteria and promote skin healing. Its ability to draw moisture into the skin makes it ideal for hydration and helping the skin maintain its natural glow. When combined with oatmeal, honey enhances the exfoliant's ability to cleanse and hydrate the skin while promoting overall skin health.

Variations and Additions:

- **Oatmeal, Honey, and Yogurt Exfoliant**: Add a tablespoon of yogurt for its lactic acid, which provides gentle chemical exfoliation, leaving the skin smooth and soft.
- **Oatmeal, Honey, and Lemon Exfoliant**: Add a few drops of lemon juice for brightening benefits. Lemon's natural astringent properties help tighten pores and even out skin tone, though it should be used sparingly on sensitive skin.
- **Oatmeal, Honey, and Aloe Vera Exfoliant**: Mix in a teaspoon of aloe vera gel for added soothing and hydration, particularly for irritated or inflamed skin.
- **Oatmeal, Honey, and Cinnamon Exfoliant**: Add a pinch of cinnamon for its anti-inflammatory and acne-fighting properties. Cinnamon also boosts circulation, promoting a healthy glow.

Additional Benefits of Oatmeal and Honey Exfoliant:

- **Improves Skin Tone and Texture**: Regular use of this exfoliant helps to smooth uneven texture and improve the overall appearance of the skin by removing dead cells and revealing fresh, healthy skin underneath.
- **Reduces Acne Breakouts**: The combination of honey's antibacterial properties and oatmeal's ability to absorb excess oil makes this exfoliant an excellent choice for reducing acne and preventing future breakouts.
- **Gentle Enough for Frequent Use**: Unlike harsh chemical exfoliants, the oatmeal and honey exfoliant is gentle enough to be used 2-3 times a week without over-exfoliating or irritating the skin.
- **Minimizes the Appearance of Pores**: Oatmeal's ability to cleanse deeply, combined with honey's pore-tightening effects, helps to minimize the appearance of large pores over time.

Precautions:

- **Patch Test First**: While oatmeal and honey are generally safe for most skin types, always perform a patch test before using the exfoliant on your face to ensure there's no allergic reaction.
- **Gentle Application**: Because this is a physical exfoliant, be sure to apply it with gentle, circular motions to avoid damaging the skin. Over-scrubbing can lead to micro-tears and irritation.
- **Avoid Sun Exposure After Lemon**: If you add lemon juice to the exfoliant, be cautious about sun exposure afterward, as lemon can increase photosensitivity, leading to sunburn or skin irritation.

Chapter 8

Improving Sleep Quality

- Understanding Sleep Disorders
- Top 5 Herbal Recipes for Restful Sleep
  1. Valerian Root Sleep Tea
  2. Hops Sleep Pillow Sachet
  3. Magnolia Bark Nighttime Tonic
  4. California Poppy Relaxation Elixir
  5. Chamomile and Lavender Bedtime Tea

Understanding Sleep Disorders

Understanding Sleep Disorders is essential for recognizing how disruptions in sleep can negatively impact both physical and mental well-being. Sleep is a critical biological process that restores and repairs the body and mind, yet millions of people struggle with sleep disorders that interfere with their ability to rest properly. These conditions range from difficulty falling asleep to staying awake at the wrong times or engaging in unusual behaviors during sleep. Sleep disorders not only impair daily functioning but also contribute to a host of long-term health issues, including cardiovascular disease, depression, and weakened immune function.

The Role of Sleep in Overall Health:

Sleep is essential for maintaining numerous bodily functions, including cognitive processing, memory consolidation, muscle repair, and immune response. A regular sleep cycle, also known as the **circadian rhythm**, regulates when the body feels alert and when it feels tired. Sleep is divided into several stages, including **REM (rapid eye movement)** and **non-REM sleep**, each playing a different role in physical restoration and mental rejuvenation. Without adequate quality sleep, individuals may experience decreased cognitive performance, mood swings, and increased susceptibility to illness.

Common Sleep Disorders:

1. **Insomnia**:
   - **Symptoms**: Difficulty falling asleep, waking frequently during the night, or waking up too early and being unable to return to sleep. Insomnia can be short-term (acute) or long-term (chronic).
   - **Causes**: Stress, anxiety, depression, irregular sleep schedules, poor sleep hygiene, or underlying medical conditions.
   - **Effects**: Daytime fatigue, irritability, difficulty concentrating, and increased risk of depression or anxiety.

2. **Sleep Apnea**:
   - **Symptoms**: Loud snoring, pauses in breathing, gasping for air during sleep, and excessive daytime sleepiness.
   - **Causes**: Obstructive sleep apnea (OSA) occurs when the muscles in the throat relax and block the airway, while central sleep apnea is caused by the brain's failure to signal proper breathing.
   - **Effects**: Poor sleep quality, increased risk of high blood pressure, heart disease, stroke, and metabolic disorders.

3. **Restless Legs Syndrome (RLS)**:
   - **Symptoms**: Uncomfortable sensations in the legs, often described as tingling or burning, with an irresistible urge to move them, especially at night.
   - **Causes**: RLS can be linked to iron deficiency, chronic diseases such as kidney failure, or neurological issues.

Ch. 8 - Improving Sleep Quality

- **Effects**: Disrupted sleep, leading to fatigue, reduced quality of life, and impaired concentration during the day.

4. **Narcolepsy**:

   - **Symptoms**: Sudden and uncontrollable episodes of sleep during the day, sometimes accompanied by **cataplexy**, a sudden loss of muscle control triggered by strong emotions.
   - **Causes**: Narcolepsy is a neurological disorder caused by a deficiency in **hypocretin**, a brain chemical that regulates wakefulness.
   - **Effects**: Inability to stay awake, difficulty sleeping at night, and a profound impact on daily functioning and safety (e.g., driving).

5. **Circadian Rhythm Disorders**:

   - **Symptoms**: Misalignment between the body's internal clock and the environment, resulting in difficulty falling asleep at desired times (e.g., delayed sleep phase disorder) or trouble staying awake during the day.
   - **Causes**: Shift work, jet lag, irregular schedules, or biological factors.
   - **Effects**: Chronic fatigue, reduced productivity, and impaired concentration.

6. **Parasomnias**:

   - **Symptoms**: Unusual behaviors during sleep, such as sleepwalking, night terrors, sleep talking, or **REM sleep behavior disorder**, where individuals physically act out their dreams.
   - **Causes**: Stress, trauma, certain medications, or underlying neurological disorders.
   - **Effects**: Sleep disruptions, potential injury, and embarrassment or confusion upon waking.

Factors Contributing to Sleep Disorders:

- **Lifestyle Choices**: Poor sleep hygiene, such as inconsistent bedtimes, excessive use of electronic devices before sleep, and consumption of caffeine, alcohol, or nicotine, can lead to disrupted sleep.
- **Mental Health**: Anxiety, depression, and stress are closely linked to insomnia and other sleep disturbances, creating a cycle where poor sleep worsens mental health issues, and vice versa.
- **Medical Conditions**: Chronic pain, respiratory issues, gastrointestinal disorders, and neurological conditions like Parkinson's disease can significantly interfere with sleep quality.
- **Aging**: As people age, sleep patterns naturally change, often leading to lighter, more fragmented sleep. Older adults are more prone to insomnia and other sleep-related issues like sleep apnea or restless legs syndrome.

The Impact of Sleep Disorders on Health:

- **Physical Health**: Chronic sleep deprivation is associated with an increased risk of developing serious health conditions such as obesity, diabetes, cardiovascular disease, and a weakened immune system. Sleep disorders, particularly sleep apnea, significantly raise the risk of heart attacks and strokes due to frequent drops in oxygen levels during sleep.

- **Mental Health**: Sleep disorders can exacerbate anxiety, depression, and stress, as sleep is essential for emotional regulation. Inadequate sleep is also linked to increased irritability, mood swings, and a reduced ability to cope with stress.

- **Cognitive Function**: Lack of sleep impairs cognitive performance, leading to slower reaction times, difficulty focusing, and poor memory retention. This can affect daily activities, job performance, and even increase the likelihood of accidents.

Diagnosing Sleep Disorders:

To accurately diagnose a sleep disorder, healthcare providers may use several methods:

- **Sleep Diary**: Patients may be asked to record their sleep patterns, habits, and any symptoms they experience over several weeks.

- **Polysomnography (Sleep Study)**: This test involves monitoring brain waves, breathing, heart rate, and other factors during sleep to detect disorders like sleep apnea or parasomnias.

- **Multiple Sleep Latency Test (MSLT)**: This test measures how quickly someone falls asleep during the day and is often used to diagnose narcolepsy.

Treatment and Management of Sleep Disorders:

1. **Improving Sleep Hygiene**: Establishing a consistent sleep schedule, creating a calming bedtime routine, limiting screen time, and ensuring a comfortable sleep environment can help regulate sleep patterns and improve sleep quality.

2. **Cognitive Behavioral Therapy for Insomnia (CBT-I)**: CBT-I is an effective, non-pharmaceutical treatment that helps individuals change unhelpful thoughts and behaviors that contribute to insomnia.

3. **Medications and Devices**:
    - For sleep apnea, **CPAP (continuous positive airway pressure)** therapy is used to keep airways open during sleep.
    - Medications may be prescribed to manage insomnia, RLS, or narcolepsy, though they are usually a short-term solution.

4. **Treating Underlying Conditions**: Addressing medical conditions like chronic pain or mental health issues can improve sleep disorders associated with these problems.

5. **Melatonin Supplements**: For circadian rhythm disorders, melatonin may be prescribed to help regulate sleep-wake cycles, especially in cases of shift work or jet lag.

Top 5 Herbal Recipes for Restful Sleep

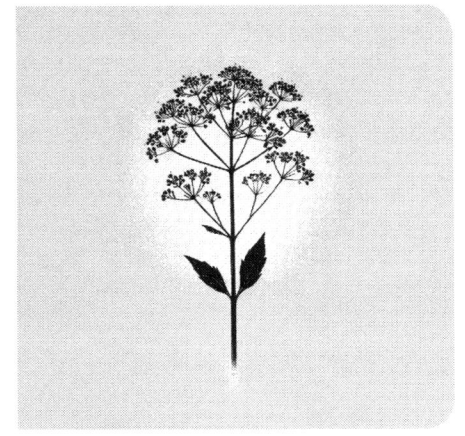

1. Valerian Root Sleep Tea

Valerian Root Sleep Tea is a natural herbal remedy known for its ability to promote relaxation and improve sleep quality. Valerian root (*Valeriana officinalis*) has been used for centuries as a mild sedative and sleep aid in traditional medicine. This tea is particularly beneficial for individuals suffering from insomnia, anxiety, or restless sleep. By calming the nervous system and easing tension, valerian root tea helps induce a state of relaxation, making it easier to fall asleep and stay asleep throughout the night.

Key Benefits of Valerian Root Sleep Tea:

- **Promotes Relaxation**: Valerian root contains compounds like **valerenic acid** and **iridoids**, which have been shown to interact with the brain's GABA receptors, promoting a calming effect and reducing nervous tension. This makes it ideal for those dealing with stress or anxiety.
- **Improves Sleep Quality**: Regular consumption of valerian root tea can help individuals fall asleep faster and enjoy deeper, more restorative sleep. Its sedative properties are particularly effective for those with insomnia or frequent nighttime awakenings.
- **Reduces Anxiety and Stress**: Valerian root has mild anxiolytic properties, making it a natural remedy for anxiety and stress. It helps reduce mental chatter and physical restlessness, allowing the body to relax.
- **Eases Muscle Tension**: The soothing properties of valerian root can help relax tense muscles, which is particularly helpful for individuals who suffer from physical discomfort that disrupts their sleep.
- **Non-Habit Forming**: Unlike some prescription sleep aids, valerian root is non-habit forming, making it a safe and natural alternative for those looking to improve their sleep without dependency.

How to Make Valerian Root Sleep Tea:

Ingredients:
- 1/2 cup puredried valerian root (or a valerian root tea bag)
- 1 cup boiling water
- Optional: 1 teaspoon honey (for sweetness)
- Optional: 1-2 drops lavender or chamomile essential oil (fsoothing properties)

Instructions:

1. In a teapot or mug, place 1 teaspoon of dried valerian root or a valerian root tea bag.
2. Pour 1 cup of boiling water over the valerian root and allow it to steep for 10-15 minutes, ensuring the active compounds are fully extracted.
3. If desired, add 1 teaspoon of honey to sweeten the tea and a few drops of lavender or chamomile essential oil to enhance the calming effects.
4. Strain the valerian root (if using loose herbs) and sip the tea about 30-60 minutes before bed for optimal relaxation and sleep benefits.

How to Use:

- **As a Nightly Sleep Aid**: Drink a cup of valerian root sleep tea approximately 30-60 minutes before bedtime to help prepare your body and mind for sleep.

- **For Stress Relief**: On particularly stressful days, you can enjoy valerian root tea earlier in the evening to promote relaxation and ease into a calm state.

Science Behind Valerian Root's Benefits for Sleep:

Valerian root's primary action on the nervous system is due to its ability to increase levels of **gamma-aminobutyric acid (GABA)**, a neurotransmitter that promotes relaxation and reduces anxiety. Low levels of GABA are often linked to sleep disorders, including insomnia and anxiety. Studies published in *Phytotherapy Research* have shown that valerian root can enhance GABA's sedative effects, allowing individuals to fall asleep faster and enjoy a more restful sleep.

Additionally, valerian root's active compounds, such as **valerenic acid** and **isovaleric acid**, have been found to inhibit the breakdown of GABA in the brain, further contributing to its calming effects. These compounds also have a mild sedative impact, making valerian root tea an effective remedy for improving sleep quality without the risk of morning drowsiness.

Variations and Additions:

- **Valerian and Chamomile Sleep Tea**: Combine valerian root with chamomile flowers for a soothing blend that enhances relaxation and helps reduce anxiety. Chamomile also adds a mild, pleasant flavor.
- **Valerian and Lavender Sleep Tea**: Add dried lavender flowers to the tea for a calming aroma and additional sleep-promoting benefits. Lavender's relaxing properties complement valerian root's sedative effects.
- **Valerian and Lemon Balm Sleep Tea**: Lemon balm is known for its calming and mood-enhancing effects. Mix it with valerian root to create a tea that supports relaxation and relieves stress-induced insomnia.

- **Valerian and Peppermint Sleep Tea**: For a refreshing twist, add dried peppermint leaves. Peppermint helps soothe digestion, which can be beneficial for those whose sleep is affected by digestive discomfort.

Additional Benefits of Valerian Root Sleep Tea:

- **Reduces Nighttime Restlessness**: Valerian root tea helps calm both the mind and body, reducing physical restlessness and mental overactivity that can prevent restful sleep.
- **Supports Emotional Well-Being**: By reducing stress and anxiety, valerian root tea helps create emotional balance, which can improve overall mental health and promote better sleep.
- **May Help with Headaches**: Valerian root's muscle-relaxing properties can help relieve tension headaches, which are often linked to stress and poor sleep.
- **Natural Menopause Relief**: Valerian root has been shown to help alleviate symptoms of menopause, such as hot flashes and sleep disturbances, providing relief for women going through this life stage.

Precautions:

- **Possible Drowsiness**: While valerian root tea is non-habit forming, it can cause drowsiness in some individuals. Avoid drinking valerian root tea during the day or before engaging in activities that require alertness, such as driving.
- **Consult with a Doctor**: If you are pregnant, breastfeeding, or taking prescription medications (especially sedatives or anti-anxiety medications), consult your healthcare provider before using valerian root tea.
- **Mild Side Effects**: Some people may experience mild side effects such as headaches, dizziness, or digestive discomfort. Start with a small dose to see how your body responds.

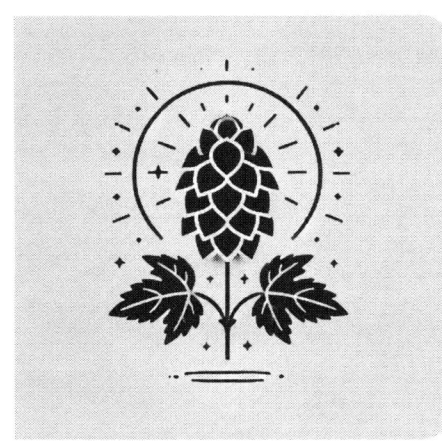

2. Hops Sleep Pillow Sachet

Hops Sleep Pillow Sachet is a natural remedy designed to promote relaxation and enhance sleep quality. Derived from the dried flowers of the *Humulus lupulus* plant, commonly known as hops, this sleep aid works by releasing a mild, calming scent that helps ease stress and tension, making it easier to fall asleep. Hops have been used for centuries for their sedative properties, particularly in combination with other calming herbs. By placing a hops sachet inside your pillow or near your bed, you can enjoy a gentle, soothing aroma that supports a restful night's sleep.

Key Benefits of Hops Sleep Pillow Sachet:

- **Promotes Relaxation**: Hops contain compounds like **methylbutenol**, which have mild sedative effects. These compounds help calm the nervous system, reduce restlessness, and promote relaxation, making it easier to fall asleep.
- **Improves Sleep Quality**: The aroma released by hops can help enhance sleep quality by promoting deeper, more restorative sleep. This makes hops especially beneficial for those with difficulty staying asleep or experiencing frequent nighttime awakenings.
- **Eases Anxiety and Stress**: The calming scent of hops helps reduce anxiety and tension, which are common contributors to insomnia. Using a hops sachet before bed can create a relaxing environment that eases both physical and mental stress.
- **Natural Sleep Aid**: Unlike prescription sleep medications, hops are a natural, non-habit-forming remedy. They provide gentle, safe support for sleep without causing grogginess or dependence.
- **Complements Other Relaxing Herbs**: Hops pair well with other calming herbs like lavender or chamomile, enhancing their combined effects to promote a more peaceful sleep experience.

How to Make a Hops Sleep Pillow Sachet:

Ingredients:

- 1/2 cup dried hops flowers
- Optional: 1/4 cup dried lavender flowers (for added relaxation)
- Optional: 1/4 cup dried chamomile flowers (for calming and sleep support)
- Small cotton or muslin sachet bag

Instructions:

1. Combine 1/2 cup of dried hops flowers with your choice of other relaxing herbs, such as 1/4 cup of dried lavender or chamomile, in a small bowl.
2. Mix the herbs gently to combine their fragrances.
3. Spoon the herbal mixture into a small cotton or muslin sachet bag, securing it tightly.
4. Place the sachet inside your pillowcase or on your bedside table to enjoy the calming effects of the hops and herbs as you sleep.

How to Use:

- **For Sleep**: Place the hops sachet inside your pillowcase or next to your pillow before bed. The gentle aroma will be released throughout the night, helping to calm your mind and promote relaxation.

• **For Relaxation**: Use the sachet in the evening while unwinding or meditating to help reduce stress and prepare your body for sleep.

Science Behind Hops' Benefits for Sleep:

Hops contain **volatile oils** and compounds like **humulone** and **lupulone**, which are responsible for their sedative effects. Research published in the *Journal of Phytotherapy Research* indicates that these compounds help calm the central nervous system, making hops an effective natural remedy for insomnia and anxiety. Hops work by interacting with GABA (gamma-aminobutyric acid) receptors in the brain, which play a role in promoting relaxation and reducing nervous system activity.

The soothing scent of hops, especially when combined with other relaxing herbs like lavender, has been found to reduce sleep latency (the time it takes to fall asleep) and improve overall sleep quality. Hops are also commonly used in herbal sleep formulas, such as valerian-hops combinations, which have been shown to effectively promote relaxation without causing morning drowsiness.

Variations and Additions:

• **Hops and Lavender Sachet**: Add dried lavender flowers to the hops for a floral, calming aroma. Lavender is well-known for its ability to reduce stress and improve sleep quality, making this combination ideal for a restful night.

• **Hops and Chamomile Sachet**: Chamomile's calming properties complement the sedative effects of hops. This variation is perfect for those seeking a gentle, soothing blend to ease tension and promote sleep.

• **Hops and Rose Petal Sachet**: For a touch of luxury, add dried rose petals to the hops. Rose petals not only enhance the fragrance but also have mild relaxing effects, making this sachet both beautiful and effective.

• **Hops and Lemon Balm Sachet**: Lemon balm's mild sedative effects can enhance the calming properties of hops. This combination is excellent for relieving stress and anxiety while promoting better sleep.

Additional Benefits of Hops Sleep Pillow Sachet:

• **Promotes Calmness Throughout the Night**: The continuous release of hops' aroma during the night helps maintain a calm, restful environment, reducing the likelihood of waking up due to stress or anxiety.

• **Safe and Non-Toxic**: Hops are a natural, non-toxic herb that provides a safe alternative to sleep medications. It can be used nightly without risk of dependence or adverse side effects.

• **Portable and Convenient**: The sachet is easy to carry, allowing you to bring it along during travel or stressful times to maintain your sleep routine.

• **Natural Air Freshener**: In addition to promoting sleep, the hops sachet doubles as a natural air freshener, adding a pleasant, calming scent to your bedroom.

Precautions:

• **Mild Allergic Reactions**: While rare, some individuals may experience mild allergic reactions to hops. If you notice any irritation or discomfort, discontinue use.

• **Replace Regularly**: Hops sachets can lose their effectiveness over time as the essential oils evaporate. To maintain the potency of the scent, replace the sachet every few months or refresh it with a few drops of lavender or chamomile essential oil.

• **Avoid Ingestion**: The hops sachet is meant for external use only. While hops are safe for consumption in small amounts (e.g., in teas), they should not be ingested directly from the sachet.

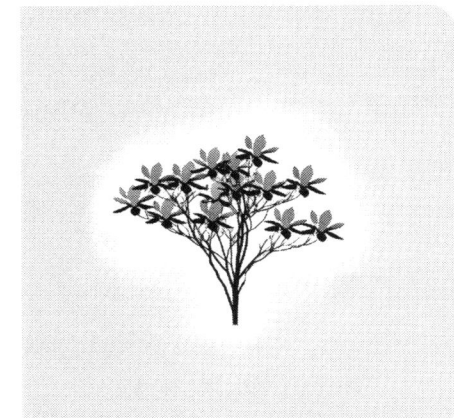

3. Magnolia Bark Nighttime Tonic

Magnolia Bark Nighttime Tonic is a natural remedy crafted from the bark of the *Magnolia officinalis* tree, renowned for its calming and sedative properties. For centuries, magnolia bark has been used in traditional Chinese medicine to promote relaxation, reduce anxiety, and improve sleep quality. This tonic is particularly beneficial for individuals experiencing stress-related insomnia, frequent nighttime awakenings, or trouble falling asleep. Magnolia bark works by supporting the nervous system and helping the body and mind relax, making it easier to drift into a peaceful and restorative sleep.

Key Benefits of Magnolia Bark Nighttime Tonic:

- **Promotes Deep Sleep**: Magnolia bark contains **honokiol** and **magnolol**, compounds that have been shown to promote sleep by interacting with GABA receptors in the brain, helping to induce calmness and relaxation. This makes it easier to fall asleep and enjoy uninterrupted, deep sleep.
- **Reduces Anxiety and Stress**: Magnolia bark's anxiolytic (anti-anxiety) properties help reduce feelings of stress and worry, making it particularly effective for those who experience sleep disturbances due to mental tension or anxiety.
- **Balances Cortisol Levels**: Research suggests that magnolia bark can help regulate cortisol, the stress hormone, particularly at night. By balancing cortisol levels, magnolia bark helps reduce nighttime anxiety and allows the body to enter a restful state more easily.
- **Supports Relaxation**: The calming effects of magnolia bark help ease physical tension and relax the muscles, which can contribute to a more comfortable and restful sleep experience.
- **Non-Habit Forming**: Unlike pharmaceutical sleep aids, magnolia bark is a natural remedy that promotes sleep without causing dependency or morning drowsiness. It offers a gentle, non-invasive way to improve sleep patterns.

How to Make Magnolia Bark Nighttime Tonic:

Ingredients:
- 1 teaspoon dried magnolia bark (available in health food stores or online)
- 1 cup water
- Optional: 1 teaspoon honey (for sweetness)
- Optional: 1 teaspoon chamomile flowers (for added relaxation)
- Optional: 1-2 drops lavender essential oil (for extra calming effects)

Instructions:

1. In a small saucepan, bring 1 cup of water to a gentle simmer.
2. Add 1 teaspoon of dried magnolia bark and, if desired, 1 teaspoon of chamomile flowers.
3. Let the mixture simmer for 10-15 minutes to extract the beneficial compounds from the magnolia bark.
4. Remove from heat and strain the tonic into a cup.
5. If desired, stir in 1 teaspoon of honey for sweetness and add a drop or two of lavender essential oil for enhanced calming effects.
6. Sip the tonic about 30-60 minutes before bed to promote relaxation and prepare your body for sleep.

How to Use:

- **For Sleep**: Drink one cup of magnolia bark nighttime tonic 30-60 minutes before bed to help calm the mind and prepare for a restful night's sleep.
- **For Stress Relief**: On particularly stressful evenings, enjoy the tonic earlier to promote relaxation and ease tension.

Science Behind Magnolia Bark's Benefits for Sleep:

Magnolia bark's primary active compounds, **honokiol** and **magnolol**, have been shown to interact with **GABA receptors** in the brain, the same receptors that are targeted by pharmaceutical sedatives. GABA is a neurotransmitter that helps inhibit neural activity, promoting relaxation and reducing stress. By enhancing GABA's activity, magnolia bark helps reduce anxiety, quiet mental chatter, and prepare the body for sleep.

In addition to its effects on GABA, magnolia bark also plays a role in regulating **cortisol**, a hormone that can spike during periods of stress. Elevated cortisol levels at night can disrupt sleep by increasing alertness and anxiety. Magnolia bark has been found to lower cortisol, particularly during the nighttime, which can help individuals with stress-related sleep issues.

Research published in the *Journal of Ethnopharmacology* has demonstrated magnolia bark's potential as a natural sleep aid, showing that it can reduce the time it takes to fall asleep, improve sleep quality, and reduce the frequency of nighttime awakenings.

Variations and Additions:

- **Magnolia Bark and Chamomile Tonic**: Combine magnolia bark with chamomile flowers to enhance the tonic's relaxing effects. Chamomile is known for its calming properties and pairs well with magnolia bark for a soothing bedtime drink.
- **Magnolia Bark and Lemon Balm Tonic**: Lemon balm is another herb known for its ability to reduce stress and anxiety. Adding it to the tonic can further enhance its calming properties, making it perfect for those who need additional help unwinding at night.
- **Magnolia Bark and Honey Tonic**: Honey not only adds sweetness but also has mild sedative properties of its own, making it a great addition to the tonic for a more soothing experience.
- **Magnolia Bark and Valerian Root Tonic**: For individuals with severe insomnia, combining magnolia bark with valerian root can provide a stronger sedative effect. Valerian root is well-known for its sleep-inducing properties and complements magnolia bark's effects.

Additional Benefits of Magnolia Bark Nighttime Tonic:

- **Reduces Nighttime Anxiety**: Magnolia bark helps calm the mind and reduce racing thoughts, which can prevent falling asleep or staying asleep. By lowering nighttime anxiety, this tonic can help create a more peaceful sleep environment.
- **Supports Emotional Balance**: By reducing stress and regulating cortisol, magnolia bark can help improve mood and emotional resilience, promoting a greater sense of well-being during the day.
- **Improves Sleep Onset**: Magnolia bark helps individuals fall asleep faster by promoting relaxation and reducing the time it takes to transition from wakefulness to sleep.
- **May Help with Menopause Symptoms**: Magnolia bark is sometimes used to help alleviate sleep disturbances and mood changes associated with menopause, such as night sweats and insomnia.

Precautions:

- **Mild Side Effects**: While magnolia bark is generally considered safe, some individuals may experience mild side effects such as dizziness or gastrointestinal discomfort. Start with a small dose to see how your body responds.
- **Consult with a Doctor**: If you are pregnant, breastfeeding, or taking prescription medications (particularly sedatives or anti-anxiety medications), consult your healthcare provider before using magnolia bark tonic.
- **Avoid Overuse**: Although non-habit forming, it's important to use magnolia bark in moderation. Continuous, excessive use may lead to excessive sedation during the day.

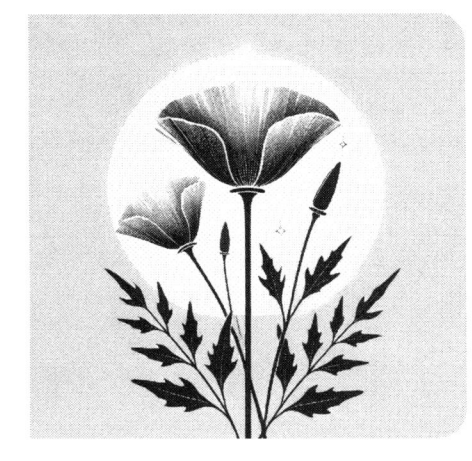

4. California Poppy Relaxation Elixir

California Poppy Relaxation Elixir is a natural herbal remedy made from the *Eschscholzia californica* plant, commonly known as the California poppy. Known for its gentle sedative and calming properties, California poppy has been used for centuries in traditional medicine to promote relaxation, reduce anxiety, and improve sleep. This elixir is particularly helpful for those who experience stress, anxiety, or insomnia, offering a non-addictive and safe way to calm the nervous system. By easing mental and physical tension, California poppy helps create a state of relaxation, making it an excellent choice for unwinding before bedtime or managing daily stress.

Key Benefits of California Poppy Relaxation Elixir:

- **Promotes Relaxation**: California poppy contains natural alkaloids like **protopine** and **cryptopine**, which have mild sedative effects. These compounds work to calm the nervous system, helping to reduce restlessness and tension, making it easier to relax.
- **Reduces Anxiety and Stress**: This elixir is particularly effective for those who struggle with anxiety or high levels of stress. California poppy helps soothe racing thoughts and anxiety, encouraging a calmer state of mind.
- **Supports Better Sleep**: California poppy has long been used to treat insomnia and other sleep disturbances. It helps individuals fall asleep more easily and stay asleep longer by promoting relaxation and reducing nighttime anxiety.
- **Eases Muscle Tension**: In addition to its calming effects on the mind, California poppy also has muscle-relaxing properties, making it beneficial for those who experience physical tension or discomfort that can interfere with relaxation.
- **Non-Habit Forming**: Unlike many pharmaceutical sleep aids or anti-anxiety medications, California poppy is a non-addictive, gentle alternative that can be used regularly without the risk of dependence or grogginess.

How to Make California Poppy Relaxation Elixir:

Ingredients:

- 1 tablespoon dried California poppy (or 2-3 fresh California poppy flowers, if available)
- 1 cup water
- 1 teaspoon honey (optional, for sweetness)
- Optional: 1 teaspoon dried chamomile flowers (for added relaxation)
- Optional: 1/2 teaspoon lemon balm (for additional calming effects)

Instructions:

1. In a small saucepan, bring 1 cup of water to a gentle boil.
2. Add 1 tablespoon of dried California poppy (or the fresh flowers, if using) and, if desired, chamomile or lemon balm for extra calming properties.
3. Reduce heat and let the mixture simmer for 10-15 minutes to extract the medicinal compounds from the California poppy.
4. Remove from heat, strain the mixture into a cup, and stir in 1 teaspoon of honey if you prefer a sweetened elixir.
5. Drink the elixir about 30-60 minutes before bedtime or during periods of stress for relaxation and calm.

How to Use:

- **For Relaxation**: Drink one cup of California poppy relaxation elixir when feeling stressed or anxious to calm the mind and body.
- **For Sleep**: Enjoy the elixir about 30-60 minutes before bed to promote restful sleep and reduce nighttime anxiety.

Science Behind California Poppy's Benefits:

The calming effects of California poppy are largely due to its active compounds, including **protopine**, **cryptopine**, and other alkaloids. These compounds interact with the brain's **GABA receptors**, which regulate neural excitability and promote a state of calm. By enhancing GABA activity, California poppy helps inhibit overactive brain signals, reducing anxiety and promoting relaxation.

Research published in the *Journal of Ethnopharmacology* has shown that California poppy has mild sedative and anxiolytic (anti-anxiety) properties, making it an effective natural remedy for both insomnia and anxiety. Its muscle-relaxing effects further enhance its ability to ease tension and support restful sleep without causing dependency or morning grogginess.

Variations and Additions:

- **California Poppy and Chamomile Elixir**: Adding chamomile to the elixir enhances its calming effects, as chamomile is well-known for its ability to promote relaxation and improve sleep.
- **California Poppy and Lemon Balm Elixir**: Lemon balm, with its mild sedative and stress-relieving properties, pairs perfectly with California poppy to create an even more powerful relaxation elixir.
- **California Poppy and Lavender Elixir**: Add dried lavender flowers to the elixir for a soothing floral aroma and additional calming benefits. Lavender is known for its ability to reduce anxiety and promote relaxation.
- **California Poppy and Passionflower Elixir**: Passionflower is another powerful herb that promotes relaxation and helps manage anxiety. Combining it with California poppy creates a potent elixir for those who need extra support for stress relief.

Additional Benefits of California Poppy Relaxation Elixir:

- **Helps with Mild Pain Relief**: California poppy's mild analgesic properties make it useful for easing tension headaches or minor aches and pains, further contributing to relaxation.
- **Balances Mood**: By reducing anxiety and stress, this elixir can help balance mood and support emotional well-being, making it a useful tool for managing the ups and downs of daily life.
- **Improves Sleep Quality**: California poppy not only helps with falling asleep but also improves the quality of sleep by promoting longer, deeper sleep cycles.
- **Calms Hyperactivity**: This elixir is gentle enough to use for children who struggle with restlessness or hyperactivity, helping to calm the nervous system naturally.

Precautions:

- **Avoid During Pregnancy**: California poppy should not be used by pregnant or breastfeeding women, as its effects on pregnancy are not well studied.
- **Mild Side Effects**: Although rare, some individuals may experience mild side effects such as dizziness or drowsiness during the day. It's best to start with a small dose and see how your body responds.
- **Consult with a Doctor**: If you are taking prescription medications, especially sedatives or anti-anxiety medications, consult your healthcare provider before using California poppy to avoid potential interactions.

130. Ch. 8 - Top 5 Herbal Recipes for Restful Sleep

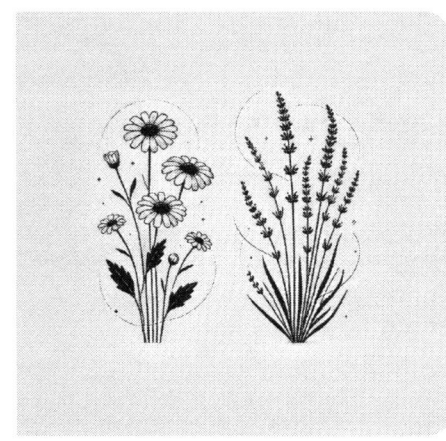

5. Chamomile and Lavender Bedtime Tea

Chamomile and Lavender Bedtime Tea is a soothing herbal blend that promotes relaxation and helps prepare the body and mind for restful sleep. Chamomile (*Matricaria chamomilla*) and lavender (*Lavandula angustifolia*) are both renowned for their calming properties, making this tea an ideal natural remedy for those who struggle with stress, anxiety, or insomnia. The gentle combination of these two herbs creates a tea that calms the nervous system, relaxes muscles, and reduces mental tension, making it easier to unwind and enjoy a peaceful night's sleep.

Key Benefits of Chamomile and Lavender Bedtime Tea:

- **Promotes Relaxation**: Chamomile contains **apigenin**, a natural compound that binds to receptors in the brain, promoting relaxation and reducing anxiety. Lavender's soothing scent and mild sedative properties help further calm the mind, making this tea perfect for winding down before bed.
- **Improves Sleep Quality**: Regular consumption of chamomile and lavender tea can help individuals fall asleep faster and enjoy deeper, more restorative sleep. Both herbs are known to gently calm the nervous system, making them ideal for treating insomnia and restlessness.
- **Reduces Anxiety and Stress**: Chamomile and lavender are both natural anxiolytics, meaning they reduce anxiety without causing drowsiness or dependence. Drinking this tea helps ease mental tension, reducing stress-related sleep disturbances.
- **Eases Muscle Tension**: Chamomile's mild anti-inflammatory and muscle-relaxing effects help ease physical tension, making it easier for the body to relax. Lavender's calming properties further contribute to a feeling of physical ease.
- **Supports Digestion**: Chamomile is known for its ability to soothe the digestive system, making this tea helpful for those who experience indigestion or bloating, which can interfere with sleep.

How to Make Chamomile and Lavender Bedtime Tea:

Ingredients:
- 1 teaspoon dried chamomile flowers
- 1/2 teaspoon dried lavender flowers
- 1 cup boiling water
- Optional: 1 teaspoon honey (for sweetness)
- Optional: 1-2 drops of vanilla extract (for added flavor)

Instructions:

1. In a teapot or mug, combine 1 teaspoon of dried chamomile flowers with 1/2 teaspoon of dried lavender flowers.

2. Pour 1 cup of boiling water over the herbs and let them steep for 5-10 minutes, allowing the calming properties of the chamomile and lavender to infuse the water.

3. Strain the tea into a cup, and if desired, stir in 1 teaspoon of honey for sweetness or a few drops of vanilla extract for a comforting flavor.

4. Drink the tea about 30-60 minutes before bedtime to promote relaxation and prepare your body for sleep.

How to Use:

- **For Sleep**: Drink a cup of chamomile and lavender bedtime tea about 30-60 minutes before going to bed. This gives the body enough time to absorb the calming effects of the herbs and helps ease you into sleep.
- **For Stress Relief**: This tea can also be enjoyed in the evening as a way to unwind after a stressful day, providing relaxation before heading to bed.

Science Behind Chamomile and Lavender's Benefits:

Chamomile's key compound, **apigenin**, binds to receptors in the brain that help induce sleep and reduce anxiety, working much like mild sedatives but without the risk of dependency. Research published in the *Journal of Advanced Nursing* found that chamomile significantly improves sleep quality and reduces nighttime awakenings, making it a valuable tool for those dealing with insomnia.

Lavender is known for its natural sedative effects, attributed to its essential oils, particularly **linalool** and **linalyl acetate**. Studies published in the *Journal of Evidence-Based Complementary and Alternative Medicine* have shown that lavender's calming properties improve sleep quality and reduce anxiety by enhancing the effects of GABA, a neurotransmitter that promotes relaxation.

Together, chamomile and lavender create a synergistic effect, amplifying each herb's ability to calm the mind and body, making this tea especially effective for promoting sleep.

Variations and Additions:

- **Chamomile, Lavender, and Lemon Balm Tea**: Add 1/2 teaspoon of dried lemon balm leaves for additional calming and anti-anxiety benefits. Lemon balm is known for reducing stress and improving sleep.
- **Chamomile, Lavender, and Peppermint Tea**: Add a few peppermint leaves for a refreshing flavor and digestive support. Peppermint can help soothe the stomach and relieve bloating or indigestion.
- **Chamomile, Lavender, and Rose Petal Tea**: Rose petals add a delicate floral flavor to the tea while offering additional calming properties, making this blend perfect for unwinding in the evening.
- **Chamomile, Lavender, and Valerian Root Tea**: For individuals with more severe insomnia, adding a small amount of valerian root enhances the sedative effects, promoting deep and restful sleep.

Additional Benefits of Chamomile and Lavender Bedtime Tea:

- **Reduces Nighttime Anxiety**: Chamomile and lavender both help calm the mind, reducing anxious thoughts that can interfere with falling asleep or staying asleep.
- **Supports Emotional Balance**: This tea promotes overall emotional well-being by reducing stress, easing tension, and creating a sense of calm before bedtime.
- **Aids Digestion**: Chamomile's soothing properties help relieve indigestion, gas, and bloating, which can be especially helpful for those who find digestive discomfort disrupts their sleep.
- **Promotes Skin Health**: Chamomile and lavender are both rich in antioxidants, which help fight free radicals and promote healthy skin, making this tea beneficial for overall wellness.

Precautions:

- **Allergic Reactions**: While rare, some individuals may be allergic to chamomile, especially those allergic to plants in the **Asteraceae** family (such as ragweed or daisies). Perform a patch test if unsure and discontinue use if you experience any allergic reactions.
- **Pregnancy**: Consult a healthcare provider before using chamomile or lavender during pregnancy, as high doses of chamomile may not be recommended.
- **Potential Drowsiness**: While this tea is meant to promote sleep, some people may feel overly drowsy or relaxed if consumed during the day. It's best reserved for nighttime use.

Chapter 9

Natural Pain Management

- Causes of Chronic and Acute Pain
- Top 5 Herbal Recipes for Pain Relief
  1. White Willow Bark Tea
  2. Turmeric and Ginger Anti-Inflammatory Shot
  3. Arnica Muscle Rub
  4. St. John's Wort Oil
  5. Devil's Claw Pain Tonic

Causes of Chronic and Acute Pain

Causes of Chronic and Acute Pain involve a variety of underlying conditions and circumstances that affect the body's tissues, nerves, and overall function. Pain is the body's way of signaling that something is wrong, but it can manifest differently depending on whether it is acute or chronic. **Acute pain** is short-term and typically occurs in response to a specific injury or illness, while **chronic pain** persists for months or even years, often outlasting the initial cause of the pain. Understanding the differences between these two types of pain, and what triggers them, is essential for effective pain management and treatment.

Acute Pain: Definition and Common Causes

Acute pain is usually sudden and sharp, lasting for a short period – from a few seconds to a few weeks – depending on the cause. This type of pain is often the result of injury or illness, and it usually subsides once the underlying cause is treated or heals.

Common causes of acute pain include:

- **Injury or Trauma**: Falls, fractures, sprains, and cuts can cause immediate pain due to tissue damage. This pain is typically intense but temporary, lasting until the injury heals.

- **Surgical Procedures**: Pain following surgery is a form of acute pain caused by tissue damage during the operation. Post-surgical pain typically diminishes as the body recovers.

- **Burns**: Burns, whether from heat, chemicals, or electricity, cause intense pain as they damage skin and underlying tissues. The severity of the pain correlates with the extent of the burn.

- **Dental Issues**: Toothaches, dental surgery, or infections such as abscesses can lead to sharp, acute pain.

- **Infections**: Acute infections, such as those caused by bacteria or viruses, can lead to localized pain, swelling, or inflammation. For example, ear infections or strep throat are common sources of acute pain.

- **Childbirth**: Labor pains are acute and intense but resolve after the birth of the baby.

Chronic Pain: Definition and Common Causes

Chronic pain persists for more than three to six months, even after the initial injury or illness that caused it has healed. This type of pain can continue long after the body has physically recovered, and in some cases, it occurs without a clear cause. Chronic pain is more complex and is often associated with ongoing health conditions or nerve damage.

Common causes of chronic pain include:

- **Arthritis**: Inflammatory conditions like osteoarthritis or rheumatoid arthritis can cause chronic joint pain due to the deterioration of cartilage or inflammation of the joints.

- **Back Pain**: Long-term back pain can be caused by injuries, spinal degeneration, herniated discs, or conditions like sciatica, which involve nerve compression.

- **Fibromyalgia**: This condition is characterized by widespread musculoskeletal pain, often accompanied by fatigue, sleep disturbances, and cognitive difficulties. The exact cause is unclear, but it is believed to involve abnormal pain processing in the brain.

- **Neuropathy**: Nerve damage or dysfunction, often associated with conditions like diabetes, can lead to chronic neuropathic pain. This type of pain is typically described as burning, tingling, or shooting.

- **Headaches**: Migraine or tension headaches can become chronic, with sufferers experiencing frequent or constant head pain that affects daily life.

- **Cancer**: Chronic pain is common in cancer patients due to tumor growth, nerve damage, or treatments like chemotherapy and radiation.

- **Chronic Inflammatory Conditions**: Conditions such as inflammatory bowel disease (IBD), which includes Crohn's disease and ulcerative colitis, cause persistent pain in the digestive tract due to inflammation.

- **Complex Regional Pain Syndrome (CRPS)**: This is a chronic pain condition that usually develops after an injury, surgery, or stroke. It is marked by prolonged, excessive pain and changes in skin color, temperature, and swelling in the affected area.

Factors Contributing to Chronic and Acute Pain:

- **Inflammation**: In both acute and chronic pain, inflammation is often a key factor. Inflammatory responses, triggered by injury or infection, cause swelling, redness, and pain as the body attempts to repair damaged tissue.

- **Nerve Damage**: When nerves are damaged, either through injury or degenerative diseases, they can misfire, sending pain signals to the brain even when there is no external cause. This is common in conditions like neuropathy or sciatica.

- **Psychological Factors**: Chronic pain can be exacerbated by psychological factors such as stress, anxiety, or depression. Pain and emotional distress often create a feedback loop, where anxiety or depression intensifies the perception of pain, and ongoing pain leads to further emotional stress.

- **Lifestyle and Posture**: Poor posture, obesity, or lack of physical activity can contribute to both acute and chronic pain, particularly in the back and joints. Sedentary lifestyles often lead to muscle weakness and joint strain, increasing the risk of chronic pain conditions.

Differences Between Chronic and Acute Pain:

- **Duration**: Acute pain is temporary, typically resolving once the underlying cause has healed, whereas chronic pain persists for months or even years, often outlasting the original cause.

- **Function**: Acute pain serves as a protective mechanism, alerting the body to injury or illness, and it usually resolves with appropriate treatment. Chronic pain, however, no longer serves a useful purpose and can become a condition in itself, disrupting a person's quality of life.

- **Treatment**: Acute pain is often treated with short-term interventions such as pain relievers (NSAIDs, acetaminophen) or rest. Chronic pain management is more complex, requiring a combination of medication, physical therapy, psychological counseling, and sometimes lifestyle changes or alternative therapies like acupuncture or massage.

Impact on Quality of Life:

- **Physical Impairment**: Chronic pain can lead to reduced mobility, making it difficult to perform daily tasks or engage in physical activity. This can contribute to muscle weakness and further pain, creating a cycle of discomfort and disability.

- **Emotional and Mental Health**: Living with chronic pain often leads to mental health challenges such as depression, anxiety, and frustration. The persistent nature of chronic pain can lead to feelings of hopelessness and isolation.

- **Sleep Disruption**: Both acute and chronic pain can interfere with sleep patterns, leading to insomnia or poor sleep quality. This can worsen pain perception and affect overall health, creating a cycle of sleep deprivation and increased pain.

Top 5 Herbal Recipes for Pain Relief

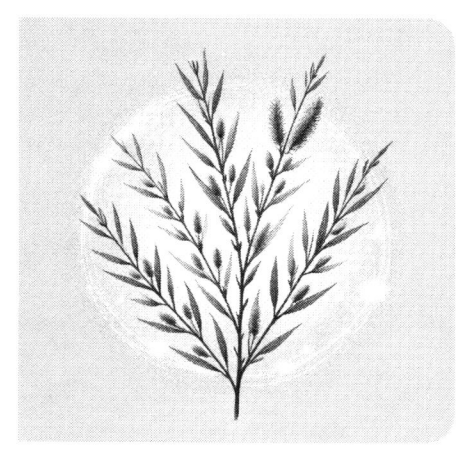

1. White Willow Bark Tea

White Willow Bark Tea is a natural remedy made from the bark of the white willow tree (*Salix alba*), known for its ability to relieve pain, reduce inflammation, and ease discomfort. White willow bark has been used for centuries in traditional medicine, dating back to ancient Greece and Egypt, where it was employed to treat fevers and pain. The active ingredient in white willow bark is **salicin**, a compound that is chemically similar to aspirin (acetylsalicylic acid). When consumed, salicin is metabolized into salicylic acid, which provides many of the same anti-inflammatory and pain-relieving benefits as aspirin, but in a gentler, more natural form.

Key Benefits of White Willow Bark Tea:

- **Pain Relief**: White willow bark is most famous for its natural analgesic (pain-relieving) properties. It is commonly used to relieve headaches, muscle pain, back pain, and joint pain, particularly in conditions like arthritis.
- **Reduces Inflammation**: The salicin in white willow bark acts as an anti-inflammatory, making it effective for reducing inflammation associated with conditions such as osteoarthritis, rheumatoid arthritis, and other inflammatory diseases.
- **Natural Alternative to Aspirin**: White willow bark offers a natural alternative to synthetic aspirin, with similar benefits but fewer side effects, particularly in terms of being gentler on the stomach. It can be used for minor aches and pains without the harshness of pharmaceuticals.
- **Eases Fever**: Like aspirin, white willow bark can help reduce fever, making it useful during colds or flu.
- **Supports Joint Health**: By reducing inflammation in the joints, white willow bark tea can help improve mobility and reduce pain in individuals suffering from joint disorders like arthritis.

How to Make White Willow Bark Tea:

Ingredients:
- 1-2 teaspoons dried white willow bark
- 1 cup water
- Optional: Honey or lemon for taste

Instructions:

1. Bring 1 cup of water to a boil.
2. Add 1-2 teaspoons of dried white willow bark to the boiling water.
3. Reduce the heat and let the bark simmer gently for 10-15 minutes.
4. Remove from heat, strain the tea, and pour it into a cup.
5. If desired, add honey or lemon for taste.
6. Drink 1-2 cups per day, depending on your needs, to help relieve pain or inflammation.

How to Use:

- **For Pain Relief**: Drink white willow bark tea 1-2 times per day to help reduce headache, muscle, or joint pain. It is particularly effective when used as a natural remedy for chronic pain conditions like arthritis or menstrual cramps.

- **For Fever or Cold Symptoms**: Drink a cup of white willow bark tea to help lower fever and ease body aches associated with colds, flu, or other illnesses.

Science Behind White Willow Bark's Benefits:

The primary active ingredient in white willow bark is **salicin**, which is metabolized into **salicylic acid** in the body. This compound has anti-inflammatory and analgesic effects similar to aspirin. Salicylic acid works by inhibiting the production of **prostaglandins**, chemicals that cause pain, inflammation, and fever. By reducing prostaglandin levels, white willow bark tea helps alleviate these symptoms.

Research published in the *Journal of Phytotherapy Research* has shown that white willow bark is effective for treating pain and inflammation, particularly in conditions like osteoarthritis. While it acts more slowly than aspirin, its effects tend to last longer, making it an excellent choice for managing chronic pain without the sharp spikes and drops often experienced with pharmaceutical pain relievers.

Variations and Additions:

- **White Willow Bark and Turmeric Tea**: Combine white willow bark with turmeric, another powerful anti-inflammatory herb. This combination is especially helpful for joint pain and inflammation caused by arthritis.
- **White Willow Bark and Ginger Tea**: Adding ginger to the tea enhances its anti-inflammatory and digestive benefits, making it a great remedy for both pain relief and digestive discomfort.
- **White Willow Bark and Chamomile Tea**: Blend with chamomile to promote relaxation and reduce stress while benefiting from white willow bark's pain-relieving properties. This combination is perfect for evening use, especially if pain interferes with sleep.

Additional Benefits of White Willow Bark Tea:

- **Fewer Side Effects**: White willow bark is gentler on the stomach than synthetic aspirin, making it a preferred choice for those who need pain relief but are sensitive to NSAIDs (non-steroidal anti-inflammatory drugs) or prone to gastrointestinal issues.
- **Supports Cardiovascular Health**: White willow bark has mild blood-thinning properties, which can help improve circulation and reduce the risk of blood clots, much like aspirin does. However, this effect is milder and should be used with caution by individuals taking blood-thinning medications.
- **May Help with Menstrual Cramps**: The anti-inflammatory and analgesic properties of white willow bark can help relieve the discomfort of menstrual cramps when taken as a tea or supplement during the menstrual cycle.
- **Improves Mobility in Arthritis**: By reducing joint inflammation, white willow bark tea helps improve mobility and ease stiffness in individuals with osteoarthritis or rheumatoid arthritis.

Precautions:

- **Aspirin Allergy**: Individuals who are allergic to aspirin or other salicylate-containing products should avoid white willow bark, as it contains salicin, which is similar to aspirin.
- **Blood Thinners**: Since white willow bark has blood-thinning effects, it should not be used by individuals taking anticoagulant medications (such as warfarin) without consulting a healthcare provider.
- **Pregnancy and Breastfeeding**: White willow bark should be avoided during pregnancy and breastfeeding, as its effects on fetal development and lactation are not fully studied.
- **Children**: Like aspirin, white willow bark should not be given to children or teenagers with viral infections, such as the flu or chickenpox, due to the risk of **Reye's syndrome**, a rare but serious condition.

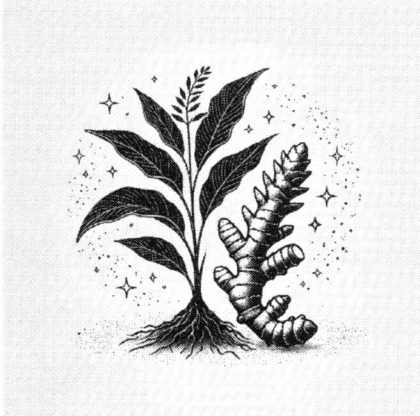

2. Turmeric and Ginger Anti-Inflammatory Shot

Turmeric and Ginger Anti-Inflammatory Shot is a potent and natural remedy designed to reduce inflammation, boost immunity, and support overall well-being. Combining two powerful anti-inflammatory ingredients, turmeric (*Curcuma longa*) and ginger (*Zingiber officinale*), this shot provides an easy and effective way to combat inflammation, promote digestion, and reduce pain. Both turmeric and ginger have been used for centuries in Ayurvedic and traditional medicine for their healing properties, making this shot a quick and concentrated way to harness their benefits.

Key Benefits of Turmeric and Ginger Anti-Inflammatory Shot:

- **Reduces Inflammation**: Turmeric contains **curcumin**, a powerful anti-inflammatory compound that helps reduce inflammation in the body by blocking certain enzymes that trigger inflammation. Ginger contains **gingerol**, which also has strong anti-inflammatory effects, making this combination highly effective in addressing inflammation associated with chronic conditions like arthritis or muscle pain.
- **Relieves Pain**: Both turmeric and ginger are natural pain relievers. This shot can help alleviate pain caused by joint inflammation, muscle soreness, or headaches by reducing the body's inflammatory response.
- **Boosts Immunity**: Turmeric and ginger both have immune-boosting properties. Curcumin in turmeric enhances the immune response, while ginger's antioxidant effects help strengthen the body's defenses against infections.
- **Aids Digestion**: Ginger is well-known for its digestive benefits, helping to soothe the stomach, relieve nausea, and reduce bloating. Combined with turmeric's ability to support gut health by reducing inflammation, this shot promotes overall digestive wellness.
- **Supports Joint Health**: By reducing inflammation and promoting circulation, this shot helps protect joints and improve mobility, making it especially beneficial for individuals with arthritis or joint discomfort.

How to Make Turmeric and Ginger Anti-Inflammatory Shot:

Ingredients:

- 1 teaspoon fresh turmeric root
(or 1/2 teaspoon ground turmeric)
- 1 teaspoon fresh ginger root
(or 1/2 teaspoon ground ginger)
- 1 tablespoon fresh lemon juice
- 1/4 teaspoon black pepper
(to enhance the absorption of curcumin)
- 1/2 teaspoon honey or maple syrup
(optional, for sweetness)
- 1/4 cup water or coconut water
(for a hydrating base)

Instructions:

1. Grate or finely chop 1 teaspoon each of fresh turmeric and ginger (or use ground versions if fresh is unavailable).
2. In a small blender or mixing bowl, combine the turmeric, ginger, lemon juice, black pepper, honey (if using), and water or coconut water.
3. Blend or whisk the mixture until well combined and smooth.
4. Strain the mixture into a small glass or shot glass to remove any pulp, and drink immediately.

How to Use:

- **For Inflammation and Pain Relief**: Take 1 shot daily, preferably in the morning, to help reduce inflammation and manage pain throughout the day.
- **For Immune Support**: Drink this shot regularly, especially during cold and flu season, to strengthen the immune system and protect against infections.

Science Behind Turmeric and Ginger's Benefits:

The primary active compound in turmeric, **curcumin**, is known for its strong anti-inflammatory and antioxidant effects. Curcumin inhibits molecules such as **cytokines** and **NF-κB**, both of which play a key role in inflammation. However, curcumin has low bioavailability, which means it is not easily absorbed by the body. This is why black pepper, which contains **piperine**, is included in the shot – it enhances curcumin absorption by up to 2,000%.

Ginger's active compound, **gingerol**, is another powerful anti-inflammatory agent. Research has shown that ginger can significantly reduce the production of pro-inflammatory markers in the body, making it effective in treating inflammation-related conditions such as osteoarthritis and muscle soreness. Studies have also demonstrated that ginger helps reduce oxidative stress, which further supports its role in protecting the body from chronic inflammation.

Variations and Additions:

- **Turmeric, Ginger, and Cinnamon Shot**: Add 1/4 teaspoon of cinnamon to the shot for additional anti-inflammatory and antioxidant benefits. Cinnamon can also help regulate blood sugar levels, making it a great addition for those seeking metabolic support.
- **Turmeric, Ginger, and Apple Cider Vinegar Shot**: Add 1 tablespoon of apple cider vinegar for digestive and detoxifying benefits. Apple cider vinegar supports gut health and balances pH levels in the body, further enhancing the benefits of turmeric and ginger.
- **Turmeric, Ginger, and Coconut Water Shot**: For hydration and electrolyte balance, use coconut water as the base. This is particularly beneficial for athletes or individuals who want a refreshing and hydrating anti-inflammatory boost.
- **Turmeric, Ginger, and Pineapple Shot**: Pineapple contains **bromelain**, an enzyme known for its anti-inflammatory and digestive benefits. Adding fresh pineapple juice to the shot creates a sweet, tropical flavor while increasing its anti-inflammatory properties.

Additional Benefits of Turmeric and Ginger Anti-Inflammatory Shot:

- **Supports Heart Health**: The anti-inflammatory properties of turmeric and ginger help reduce inflammation in the blood vessels, which may lower the risk of heart disease. Ginger also helps improve circulation, further supporting cardiovascular health.
- **Improves Skin Health**: Both turmeric and ginger are rich in antioxidants, which help fight free radicals and reduce oxidative stress in the body. This supports clearer skin and helps reduce signs of aging, such as wrinkles or dullness.
- **Promotes Detoxification**: Turmeric and ginger are known to support the liver's detoxifying processes, helping the body eliminate toxins more efficiently and improving overall metabolic health.
- **Alleviates Menstrual Cramps**: Ginger, in particular, has been shown to relieve pain associated with menstrual cramps by reducing inflammation and relaxing the muscles.

Precautions:

- **Stomach Sensitivity**: In some individuals, turmeric and ginger may cause mild digestive discomfort, especially if consumed in high doses. Start with a small amount and increase gradually if needed.
- **Blood Thinners**: Both turmeric and ginger have mild blood-thinning properties, so individuals taking anticoagulant medications (such as warfarin) or those with bleeding disorders should consult a healthcare provider before using this shot regularly.
- **Gallbladder Issues**: Turmeric may stimulate bile production, so individuals with gallbladder problems should consult their doctor before using turmeric in high doses.

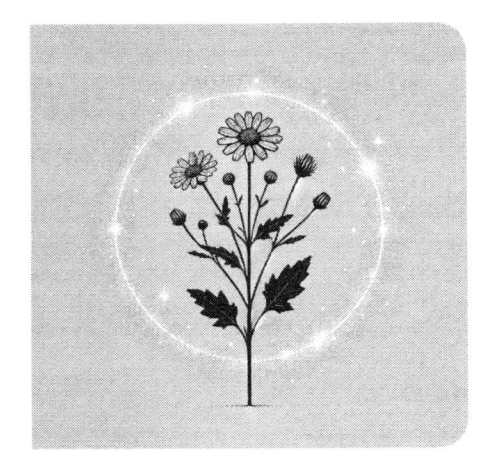

3. Arnica Muscle Rub

Arnica Muscle Rub is a topical herbal remedy made from the flowers of the *Arnica montana* plant, known for its powerful anti-inflammatory and pain-relieving properties. Arnica has been used for centuries in traditional medicine to treat muscle soreness, bruising, joint pain, and inflammation. When applied to the skin, this rub helps reduce swelling, ease muscle tension, and promote faster recovery from injuries or overuse. Arnica muscle rub is particularly beneficial for athletes, individuals recovering from physical activity, or anyone dealing with muscle aches and stiffness.

Key Benefits of Arnica Muscle Rub:

- **Reduces Muscle Soreness**: Arnica is effective at relieving muscle pain and stiffness, making it ideal for treating sore muscles after exercise, heavy lifting, or physical activity. Its anti-inflammatory properties help calm inflamed muscles and promote recovery.
- **Eases Bruising and Swelling**: Arnica is widely known for its ability to reduce bruising and swelling, making it a common remedy for soft tissue injuries, such as sprains, strains, or bumps.
- **Relieves Joint Pain**: Arnica's anti-inflammatory properties extend to joint pain, helping to reduce inflammation and discomfort associated with arthritis, tendonitis, or bursitis.
- **Improves Circulation**: When applied to the skin, arnica stimulates blood flow to the affected area, which helps speed up healing by delivering nutrients and oxygen to injured tissues.
- **Natural Pain Relief**: Arnica provides a natural, non-invasive alternative to over-the-counter pain relievers. It can be used as needed without the risk of systemic side effects like those associated with NSAIDs.

How to Make Arnica Muscle Rub:

Ingredients:
- 1/2 cup dried arnica flowers (or 1/4 cup arnica oil)
- 1/2 cup carrier oil (such as olive oil, coconut oil, or jojoba oil)
- 2 tablespoons beeswax (to solidify the rub)
- 10-15 drops essential oils (optional, such as peppermint or eucalyptus for cooling effects, or lavender for relaxation)

Instructions:

1. Infuse the oil: If you're using dried arnica flowers, begin by making an arnica-infused oil. Combine 1/2 cup dried arnica flowers with 1/2 cup carrier oil in a glass jar. Seal the jar and let it sit in a sunny windowsill for 2-3 weeks, shaking it occasionally to help the infusion process. Strain the oil through a fine mesh sieve or cheesecloth to remove the flowers.

2. Melt the beeswax: In a double boiler, gently melt 2 tablespoons of beeswax. Once melted, remove from heat.

3. Mix the oils: Stir the arnica-infused oil (or pre-made arnica oil) into the melted beeswax. Add any essential oils at this stage for additional therapeutic effects.

4. Cool and store: Pour the mixture into a small, clean jar or tin and let it cool completely. Once solidified, your arnica muscle rub is ready for use. Store the rub in a cool, dry place and use as needed.

How to Use:

5. For Muscle and Joint Pain: Massage a small amount of arnica muscle rub onto sore muscles, bruises, or achy joints 2-3 times per day or as needed. Rub gently to allow the arnica to penetrate the skin and reduce pain and swelling.

6. For Post-Workout Recovery: Apply the rub to areas of muscle tension or soreness after exercise to promote recovery and ease inflammation.

Science Behind Arnica's Benefits for Muscle and Joint Pain:

The active compounds in arnica, particularly **helenalin** and **sesquiterpene lactones**, have strong anti-inflammatory and analgesic properties. These compounds work by reducing the production of pro-inflammatory cytokines and enzymes that contribute to pain and swelling. Research published in the *Journal of Ethnopharmacology* has demonstrated that arnica is effective in reducing pain, bruising, and swelling after injuries or surgery.

Arnica also improves local blood circulation when applied to the skin, helping to speed up the healing process by increasing oxygen and nutrient delivery to the affected tissues. This makes arnica particularly useful for bruises, sprains, and muscle strains, where inflammation and tissue damage are common.

Variations and Additions:

- **Arnica and Peppermint Rub**: Add 10-15 drops of peppermint essential oil to the muscle rub for a cooling effect. Peppermint helps soothe muscle tension and provides a refreshing sensation, making it especially beneficial after intense physical activity.
- **Arnica and Lavender Rub**: Lavender essential oil can be added to the rub for its calming and anti-inflammatory properties. Lavender is ideal for easing stress-related tension or helping relax sore muscles before bed.
- **Arnica and Eucalyptus Rub**: Eucalyptus essential oil has anti-inflammatory and cooling properties that complement arnica's pain-relieving effects. This combination is great for treating joint pain or inflammation associated with arthritis.
- **Arnica and Turmeric Rub**: Add turmeric oil to the rub for enhanced anti-inflammatory effects. Turmeric's **curcumin** compounds help reduce joint and muscle inflammation, making this combination effective for chronic pain conditions like arthritis.

Additional Benefits of Arnica Muscle Rub:

Supports Faster Recovery from Injuries: Arnica helps reduce swelling and pain after injuries such as sprains, strains, or contusions, making it a popular remedy for athletes or those with physically demanding jobs.

Natural Alternative to OTC Pain Relievers: For individuals who prefer to avoid over-the-counter pain medications, arnica offers a natural solution for managing pain without systemic side effects.

Gentle on Skin: When properly prepared, arnica muscle rub is gentle enough for regular use on sore or inflamed areas without causing irritation, making it suitable for most skin types.

Anti-Bruising Properties: Arnica is well-known for reducing the appearance of bruises. By stimulating circulation and reducing inflammation, it can help fade bruises faster and alleviate the discomfort associated with them.

Precautions:

- **External Use Only**: Arnica should never be ingested or applied to open wounds, as it can be toxic when absorbed into the bloodstream. Always use arnica products externally and avoid using them on broken skin.
- **Sensitive Skin**: Some individuals may experience irritation or allergic reactions to arnica, especially if used in large amounts. Test the rub on a small area of skin first and discontinue use if irritation occurs.
- **Pregnancy and Breastfeeding**: Consult a healthcare provider before using arnica during pregnancy or breastfeeding, as its safety during these times has not been fully established.
- **Extended Use**: Arnica is most effective for short-term use. Avoid prolonged or excessive application without consulting a healthcare provider, as long-term use may lead to skin irritation.

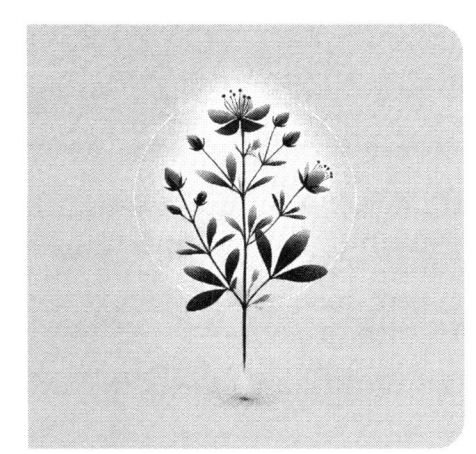

4. St. John's Wort Oil

St. John's Wort Oil is a natural topical remedy made from the flowers of *Hypericum perforatum*, known for its powerful anti-inflammatory, antiviral, and wound-healing properties. This herbal oil has been used for centuries in traditional medicine to treat skin irritations, minor burns, wounds, and nerve pain. St. John's Wort oil is particularly valued for its ability to soothe inflamed skin, relieve nerve-related discomfort, and promote faster healing of cuts and bruises. It is also used to ease the symptoms of conditions like sciatica, shingles, and minor muscle pain.

Key Benefits of St. John's Wort Oil:

- **Soothes Inflammation**: St. John's Wort oil contains **hypericin** and **hyperforin**, compounds known for their anti-inflammatory effects. When applied topically, it helps reduce swelling, redness, and irritation, making it beneficial for minor burns, sunburn, and insect bites.
- **Promotes Wound Healing**: This oil has powerful wound-healing properties, helping to speed up the repair of cuts, scrapes, and bruises. Its antimicrobial action also helps protect the skin from infection.
- **Relieves Nerve Pain**: St. John's Wort is particularly effective at easing nerve pain, including conditions like sciatica, shingles, and neuralgia. It can help soothe sharp, shooting pains and reduce discomfort from irritated nerves.
- **Reduces Muscle Pain and Cramps**: St. John's Wort oil can be massaged into sore muscles to relieve tension, muscle cramps, and mild aches, making it useful for post-exercise recovery or everyday muscle discomfort.
- **Antimicrobial and Antiviral**: In addition to its anti-inflammatory properties, St. John's Wort has antimicrobial and antiviral effects, which help protect damaged skin from infection and promote faster healing.

How to Make St. John's Wort Oil:

Ingredients:

- 1 cup fresh St. John's Wort flowers (or 1/2 cup dried flowers)
- 1 cup carrier oil (such as olive oil, jojoba oil, or almond oil)
- Clean glass jar with a lid
- Optional: 10 drops of lavender or tea tree essential oil (for additional antimicrobial benefits)

Instructions:

1. **Prepare the flowers**: If using fresh St. John's Wort flowers, gently crush or bruise the flowers to release their beneficial oils. If using dried flowers, simply measure out 1/2 cup.
2. **Infuse the oil**: Place the St. John's Wort flowers in a clean glass jar and cover them with 1 cup of carrier oil, making sure the flowers are completely submerged. Seal the jar with a tight-fitting lid.
3. **Sun infusion**: Place the jar in a sunny windowsill and let it sit for 4-6 weeks, shaking the jar every few days to help the infusion process. Over time, the oil will take on a reddish tint, indicating that the healing compounds from the flowers are being extracted.
4. **Strain the oil**: After 4-6 weeks, strain the oil through a fine mesh sieve or cheesecloth to remove the flowers. Pour the infused oil into a clean glass bottle or jar.
5. **Add essential oils** (optional): For added benefits, stir in a few drops of essential oils such as lavender or tea tree, which have antimicrobial and soothing properties.
6. **Store**: Store the St. John's Wort oil in a cool, dark place. It can last for up to a year if stored properly.

How to Use:

- **For Skin Irritations and Wounds**: Apply a small amount of St. John's Wort oil to cuts, scrapes, burns, or bruises 2-3 times daily to promote healing and reduce inflammation.
- **For Nerve Pain**: Gently massage the oil into areas affected by nerve pain, such as sciatica or shingles, to ease discomfort and calm irritated nerves.
- **For Muscle Soreness**: Rub the oil into sore muscles to relieve tension and reduce pain. It can also be used for muscle cramps and general body aches.

Science Behind St. John's Wort's Benefits:

The key active compounds in St. John's Wort – **hypericin** and **hyperforin** – are responsible for its anti-inflammatory, antimicrobial, and wound-healing properties. These compounds help reduce inflammation by inhibiting the production of pro-inflammatory cytokines, making the oil effective for treating skin irritations and mild injuries. Research published in the *Journal of Ethnopharmacology* has also highlighted St. John's Wort's ability to promote faster wound healing and protect against infections.

Hypericin is known for its mild antiviral properties, making St. John's Wort oil useful for treating viral skin conditions like cold sores or shingles. The oil's ability to soothe nerve pain is supported by its nervine properties, which help calm irritated nerves and reduce the sharp, shooting pains often associated with conditions like sciatica or neuralgia.

Variations and Additions:

- **St. John's Wort and Calendula Oil**: Combine St. John's Wort with calendula for enhanced skin-soothing and healing effects. Calendula is also excellent for treating skin irritations, burns, and rashes, making this combination ideal for sensitive or inflamed skin.
- **St. John's Wort and Lavender Oil**: Add lavender essential oil to the St. John's Wort oil for additional calming and antiseptic benefits. Lavender helps reduce inflammation and promotes relaxation, making it perfect for sore muscles or nerve pain.
- **St. John's Wort and Arnica Oil**: For stronger pain relief, combine St. John's Wort with arnica oil. Arnica is well-known for reducing bruising and easing muscle and joint pain, making this blend ideal for sports injuries or muscle strains.
- **St. John's Wort and Tea Tree Oil**: Add tea tree essential oil to the infusion for additional antimicrobial and antiseptic properties, especially useful for preventing infection in cuts, scrapes, or burns.

Additional Benefits of St. John's Wort Oil:

- **Relieves Burns and Sunburn**: St. John's Wort oil is effective at soothing and healing minor burns and sunburn. Its anti-inflammatory properties help reduce redness and pain while promoting skin repair.
- **Protects Against Infections**: The antimicrobial effects of hypericin help protect wounds from infections, making it a useful oil for cuts, abrasions, or insect bites.
- **Calms Skin Conditions**: St. John's Wort oil can be used to treat skin conditions like eczema or psoriasis by reducing inflammation and itching. It helps soothe dry, irritated skin and promotes healing.
- **Supports Emotional Well-Being**: St. John's Wort is also known for its mood-boosting properties. While the oil is primarily used topically, some believe its calming effects on the skin can extend to overall emotional well-being, helping to reduce stress and tension.

Precautions:

- **Photosensitivity**: St. John's Wort can increase skin sensitivity to sunlight. Avoid sun exposure on areas where the oil has been applied, or cover the skin with protective clothing if you will be in the sun.
- **Pregnancy and Breastfeeding**: Consult a healthcare provider before using St. John's Wort oil during pregnancy or breastfeeding, as its safety has not been fully established in these conditions.
- **Allergic Reactions**: Although rare, some individuals may experience an allergic reaction to St. John's Wort. Perform a patch test on a small area of skin before using the oil extensively to check for sensitivity or irritation.

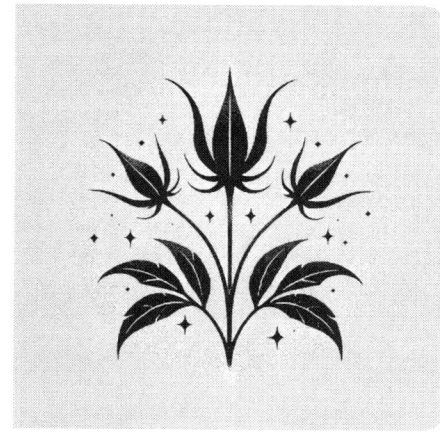

5. Devil's Claw Pain Tonic

Devil's Claw Pain Tonic is a potent natural remedy made from the root of the *Harpagophytum procumbens* plant, commonly known as devil's claw. This herb has been used in traditional African medicine for centuries to treat pain and inflammation, particularly for joint and muscle-related issues. The key active compounds in devil's claw, particularly **harpagoside**, have powerful anti-inflammatory and analgesic properties, making this tonic an excellent natural alternative for those suffering from chronic pain, arthritis, back pain, and muscle aches.

Key Benefits of Devil's Claw Pain Tonic:

- **Reduces Inflammation**: Devil's claw is known for its strong anti-inflammatory effects, particularly beneficial for conditions like osteoarthritis, rheumatoid arthritis, and other inflammatory joint disorders. It helps reduce swelling and pain in affected areas by inhibiting inflammatory markers.
- **Relieves Joint and Muscle Pain**: The analgesic properties of devil's claw make it an effective remedy for reducing pain in the joints and muscles. This tonic is especially useful for those suffering from chronic pain conditions like arthritis, lower back pain, and tendonitis.
- **Improves Mobility**: Regular use of devil's claw can help improve joint flexibility and mobility, particularly for individuals with stiff or swollen joints due to inflammation. By reducing pain and inflammation, it promotes better movement and physical function.
- **Supports Digestive Health**: In addition to its pain-relieving properties, devil's claw also aids in digestion by stimulating bile production. This can be helpful for individuals suffering from digestive issues like indigestion or bloating, often linked to poor bile flow.
- **Natural Alternative to NSAIDs**: Devil's claw provides a natural option for managing pain and inflammation without the gastrointestinal side effects often associated with long-term use of non-steroidal anti-inflammatory drugs (NSAIDs).

How to Make Devil's Claw Pain Tonic:

Ingredients:

- 1 tablespoon dried devil's claw root (or 1-2 teaspoons of devil's claw tincture)
- 1 cup water
- Optional: Honey or lemon for taste
- Optional: 1 teaspoon dried ginger root (for additional anti-inflammatory and digestive benefits)

Instructions:

1. **Boil the water**: Bring 1 cup of water to a boil.
2. **Infuse the devil's claw**: Add 1 tablespoon of dried devil's claw root (or 1-2 teaspoons of devil's claw tincture) to the boiling water.
3. **Simmer**: Reduce the heat and let the mixture simmer for 10-15 minutes to extract the beneficial compounds from the root.
4. **Strain and serve**: Strain the tonic into a cup, discarding the root pieces. If desired, add honey or lemon to improve the taste, or include dried ginger root for added benefits.
5. **Drink**: Drink the tonic once or twice daily, preferably before meals, to reduce pain and inflammation.

How to Use:

- **For Joint and Muscle Pain**: Drink 1-2 cups of devil's claw pain tonic daily to manage chronic pain and inflammation in the joints and muscles. This can be especially helpful for conditions like arthritis or back pain.

- **For Digestive Support**: Consume the tonic before meals to stimulate digestion and relieve symptoms of indigestion or bloating.

Science Behind Devil's Claw's Benefits:

The primary active ingredient in devil's claw is **harpagoside**, an iridoid glycoside that has been shown to reduce inflammation by inhibiting the production of pro-inflammatory cytokines. Research published in the *Journal of Ethnopharmacology* has demonstrated that devil's claw effectively reduces pain and inflammation in conditions such as osteoarthritis, particularly in the knee and hip joints. Studies have also shown that it can reduce lower back pain and improve mobility in individuals with chronic pain.

Harpagoside works by blocking certain enzymes, such as **cyclooxygenase (COX)** and **lipoxygenase (LOX)**, which are involved in the inflammatory process. By reducing the activity of these enzymes, devil's claw helps decrease pain and swelling in inflamed tissues, offering relief to those suffering from chronic joint and muscle pain.

Variations and Additions:

- **Devil's Claw and Ginger Tonic**: Adding ginger root to the tonic enhances its anti-inflammatory and digestive benefits. Ginger also has powerful pain-relieving properties, making this combination particularly effective for easing joint and muscle pain.
- **Devil's Claw and Turmeric Tonic**: For an even stronger anti-inflammatory effect, add 1/2 teaspoon of turmeric powder to the tonic. Turmeric contains **curcumin**, which helps further reduce inflammation and improve joint mobility.
- **Devil's Claw and Lemon Balm Tonic**: Add dried lemon balm for a calming effect. Lemon balm helps soothe nerves and muscles, making it a great addition to the tonic, especially for those who experience tension-related pain.
- **Devil's Claw and Willow Bark Tonic**: Combine with white willow bark, which contains **salicin**, a natural pain reliever similar to aspirin.

This blend offers a powerful natural remedy for managing severe pain and inflammation.

Additional Benefits of Devil's Claw Pain Tonic:

- **Supports Long-Term Joint Health**: By reducing inflammation and pain, regular use of devil's claw can help prevent further joint deterioration in conditions like osteoarthritis, improving long-term joint function and quality of life.
- **May Help with Tendonitis**: The anti-inflammatory properties of devil's claw make it useful for treating tendonitis, a condition characterized by inflammation of the tendons. It helps reduce pain and swelling, promoting faster healing.
- **Reduces Tension Headaches**: For those who suffer from tension headaches due to muscle tightness or stress, devil's claw can provide relief by relaxing tense muscles and reducing inflammation.
- **Boosts Overall Mobility**: Individuals who suffer from stiffness, especially in the morning, may find that devil's claw improves their ability to move more freely and with less pain.

Precautions:

- **Stomach Sensitivity**: While devil's claw is gentler on the stomach than NSAIDs, it may cause mild digestive upset in some individuals. If you experience stomach discomfort, consider taking it with food or reducing the dose.
- **Blood Thinners**: Devil's claw may interfere with blood-thinning medications like warfarin, as it can affect blood clotting. If you are on anticoagulants, consult a healthcare provider before using this tonic.
- **Pregnancy and Breastfeeding**: Devil's claw should be avoided during pregnancy and breastfeeding, as its safety during these periods has not been fully established.
- **Gallbladder Issues**: Devil's claw stimulates bile production, so individuals with gallbladder problems or gallstones should consult a healthcare provider before using it.

Bonus Chapter 10

The Top 10 Healing Plants Detailed Profiles

- **Introduction to Nature's Most Powerful Healers**
1. Echinacea
2. Turmeric
3. Ginger
4. Garlic
5. Lavender
6. Chamomile
7. Aloe Vera
8. Ginseng
9. Peppermint
10. Calendula

Introduction to Nature's Most Powerful Healers

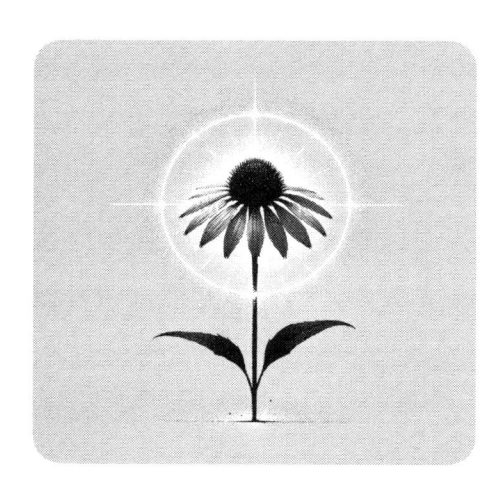

1. Echinacea

Botanical Description:

Echinacea, commonly known as purple coneflower, belongs to the *Asteraceae* family and is native to North America. The plant is easily recognized by its tall, slender stalks and striking daisy-like flowers, which come in shades of pink, purple, or white, with a prominent spiky cone at the center. There are several species of Echinacea, but the most commonly used medicinally are *Echinacea purpurea*, *Echinacea angustifolia*, and *Echinacea pallida*.

The entire plant, including its roots, flowers, and leaves, can be used for medicinal purposes, though the root is often considered the most potent part. Echinacea thrives in dry, open areas like prairies and is hardy enough to withstand a range of climates.

Healing Properties:

Echinacea is one of nature's most powerful immune modulators, primarily known for its ability to prevent and reduce the severity of respiratory infections like the common cold and flu. It works by stimulating the production and activity of white blood cells, which are essential in fighting off pathogens. Echinacea also has anti-inflammatory, antiviral, and antimicrobial properties that help the body defend itself against various infections and inflammation.

Some key healing properties of Echinacea include:

- **Boosts Immune Function**: Echinacea activates the immune system by increasing the production of immune cells, including T-cells, macrophages, and natural killer cells. This makes it particularly effective at preventing and reducing the duration of upper respiratory infections.

- **Fights Infections**: Echinacea's antimicrobial properties help the body resist bacterial and viral infections, making it useful for treating conditions such as the common cold, sinus infections, and even mild skin infections.

- **Anti-Inflammatory Effects**: Echinacea helps reduce inflammation by inhibiting certain inflammatory enzymes and pathways in the body. This makes it beneficial for easing conditions like sore throats, swollen lymph nodes, and skin irritations.

- **Antioxidant-Rich**: Echinacea contains flavonoids and phenolic compounds, which are powerful antioxidants that help protect the body from oxidative stress, reducing the risk of chronic diseases related to cell damage.

Usage Guidelines:

Echinacea can be used in various forms, including tinctures, teas, capsules, and topical creams. The most effective way to use it depends on the condition being treated and the individual's preference.

- **Tincture**: Tinctures are concentrated extracts of the herb, typically preserved in alcohol. A common dosage for preventing or treating colds and flu is 2.5 mL (about half a teaspoon) taken up to three times per day. Tinctures can be added to water or tea for easier consumption.

- **Tea**: Echinacea tea is made by steeping the dried roots, leaves, or flowers in hot water for about 10-15 minutes. It can be consumed 2-3 times a day during cold or flu season to boost immunity.

- **Capsules**: Echinacea is available in capsule form, often combined with other immune-boosting herbs like elderberry or goldenseal. Standard doses range from 300-500 mg, taken up to three times daily.

- **Topical Creams**: For skin conditions, Echinacea can be applied as a topical ointment or cream to help heal wounds, burns, or skin infections.

2. Turmeric

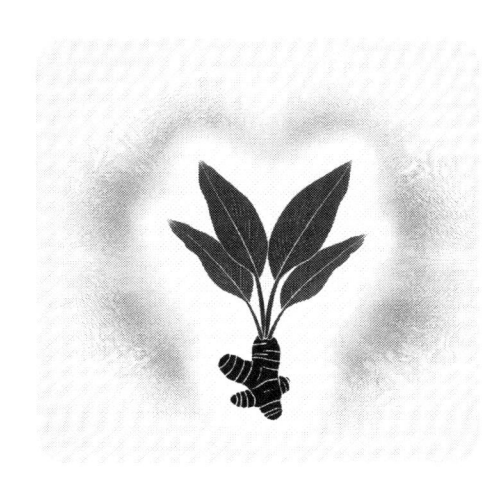

Botanical Description:

Turmeric (*Curcuma longa*) is a vibrant yellow-orange root that belongs to the *Zingiberaceae* family, which also includes ginger. Native to Southeast Asia, turmeric has been cultivated for thousands of years and is a key ingredient in Ayurvedic, traditional Chinese, and Southeast Asian medicine. The plant grows about 3 feet tall, producing large, broad leaves, with its underground rhizomes (the turmeric root) being the most valuable part for culinary and medicinal use.

The rhizome is dried and ground into the familiar golden powder used in cooking, as well as medicinal preparations. The active compound that gives turmeric its bright color and powerful health benefits is **curcumin**, a polyphenol known for its strong anti-inflammatory and antioxidant properties.

Healing Properties:

Turmeric is celebrated for its wide range of healing properties, making it one of the most potent natural remedies. Its primary active compound, curcumin, has been extensively studied for its therapeutic potential, particularly in reducing inflammation, supporting joint health, and protecting against chronic diseases.

- **Anti-Inflammatory**: Turmeric is perhaps best known for its anti-inflammatory effects. Curcumin inhibits several inflammatory molecules in the body, making turmeric an effective remedy for conditions involving chronic inflammation, such as arthritis, inflammatory bowel disease, and autoimmune disorders.

- **Antioxidant**: Curcumin is a powerful antioxidant that helps neutralize free radicals, which can damage cells and lead to chronic diseases like cancer and cardiovascular disease. It also enhances the body's own antioxidant defenses.

- **Supports Joint Health**: Due to its anti-inflammatory effects, turmeric is widely used to reduce joint pain and stiffness, particularly in individuals with osteoarthritis and rheumatoid arthritis. Studies have shown that turmeric can be as effective as nonsteroidal anti-inflammatory drugs (NSAIDs) in managing pain without the side effects.

- **Aids in Digestion**: Turmeric has long been used to improve digestion and relieve conditions like bloating, gas, and indigestion. It stimulates bile production in the liver, which aids in the digestion of fats.

- **Boosts Immune Function**: The immune-modulating effects of curcumin help strengthen the body's defenses against infections and reduce inflammation in the immune system, which is beneficial for people dealing with chronic conditions or frequent infections.

- **Heart Health**: Turmeric has cardiovascular benefits due to its ability to improve endothelial function (the lining of blood vessels), reduce cholesterol, and prevent the oxidation of LDL cholesterol, which contributes to atherosclerosis.

- **Supports Brain Health**: Curcumin has neuroprotective properties and has been studied for its potential to improve cognitive function and reduce the risk of neurodegenerative diseases like Alzheimer's. It may help by reducing brain inflammation and increasing the production of brain-derived neurotrophic factor (BDNF), a protein that supports neuron growth and function.

Usage Guidelines:

Turmeric can be consumed in a variety of forms, from the dried spice used in cooking to more concentrated extracts in supplements. Curcumin's low bioavailability (how well it is absorbed by the body) can be improved when consumed with black pepper, which contains **piperine**, a compound that enhances curcumin absorption by up to 2,000%.

- **Cooking and Spice**: Turmeric is most commonly used in cooking, especially in curries, soups, and stews. It can be sprinkled into dishes for its flavor and color, but therapeutic benefits may require more concentrated forms. Combining turmeric with black pepper and healthy fats (like coconut oil or olive oil) enhances absorption.

- **Golden Milk**: Turmeric can be made into a warm, soothing drink called golden milk, which combines turmeric powder, black pepper, ginger, and a milk of choice (often plant-based). This drink is especially good for reducing inflammation and promoting relaxation before bed.

- **Supplements**: Turmeric supplements typically contain curcumin extracts and are available in capsule or tablet form. Standard doses range from 500-2,000 mg of curcumin per day. For best results, choose a supplement that includes piperine (black pepper extract) to increase absorption.

- **Turmeric Tea**: Fresh or dried turmeric can be steeped to make a tea. To prepare, simmer fresh turmeric root or powder in water for 10 minutes, strain, and enjoy with a pinch of black pepper and honey for added flavor.

- **Topical Use**: Turmeric can also be applied topically to the skin for its anti-inflammatory and antimicrobial effects. It is often used in face masks to reduce acne, brighten the complexion, and reduce redness.

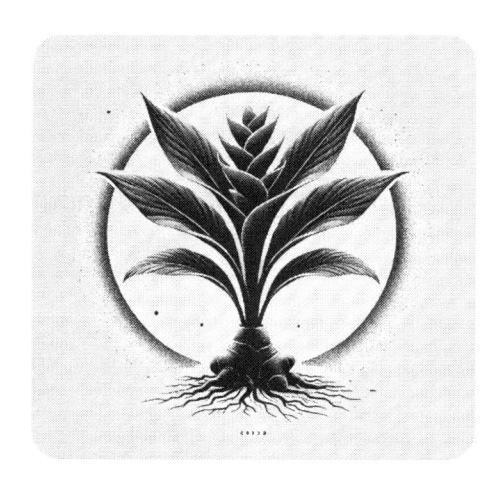

3. Ginger

Botanical Description:

Ginger (*Zingiber officinale*) is a flowering plant from the *Zingiberaceae* family, closely related to turmeric and cardamom. Native to Southeast Asia, ginger has been cultivated for thousands of years for both its culinary and medicinal uses. The part of the plant most commonly used is its rhizome, or underground stem, which is thick, knobby, and aromatic with a spicy, pungent flavor.

The ginger plant grows about 2-3 feet tall, producing narrow green leaves and yellow-green flowers. The rhizome is harvested when it reaches full maturity and can be used fresh, dried, powdered, or as an essential oil. Ginger's characteristic warmth and spicy aroma come from its high concentration of bioactive compounds, particularly **gingerol**, which is responsible for many of its therapeutic properties.

Healing Properties:

Ginger has been used in traditional medicine systems such as Ayurveda and Traditional Chinese Medicine (TCM) for centuries. Known for its wide-ranging healing properties, ginger is particularly celebrated for its digestive, anti-inflammatory, and anti-nausea effects. Modern research supports many of these traditional uses, showcasing ginger as one of nature's most powerful natural remedies.

- **Digestive Aid**: Ginger is widely known for its ability to support digestion. It stimulates digestive enzymes, increases bile production, and enhances gastric motility, helping to relieve indigestion, bloating, gas, and constipation. Ginger is particularly effective at easing nausea, whether caused by motion sickness, pregnancy (morning sickness), or chemotherapy.

- **Anti-Inflammatory**: The active compound **gingerol** has potent anti-inflammatory effects, making ginger effective for reducing inflammation throughout the body. This makes it beneficial for managing chronic inflammatory conditions such as osteoarthritis and rheumatoid arthritis, where ginger can help reduce pain and stiffness.

- **Antioxidant and Immune-Boosting**: Ginger is rich in antioxidants, which help protect cells from oxidative stress and reduce the risk of chronic diseases. Its antimicrobial and immune-boosting properties make it an effective remedy for colds, flu, and other infections, helping the body recover more quickly.

- **Pain Relief**: Ginger's anti-inflammatory effects also extend to pain relief. It can help reduce menstrual pain (dysmenorrhea) and may relieve muscle soreness and headaches, especially when consumed regularly.

- **Supports Cardiovascular Health**: Ginger has been shown to improve circulation, reduce cholesterol levels, and lower blood pressure. By reducing inflammation and improving blood flow, it helps support overall heart health and reduce the risk of cardiovascular diseases.

- **Blood Sugar Regulation**: Studies suggest that ginger can help regulate blood sugar levels, improving insulin sensitivity and lowering fasting blood glucose. This makes ginger a valuable addition to the diet for individuals managing type 2 diabetes or those looking to stabilize blood sugar levels.

Usage Guidelines:

Ginger is a versatile herb that can be used in many forms, including fresh, dried, powdered, and as an essential oil or extract. Its warm, spicy flavor pairs well with both savory and sweet dishes, and it can also be consumed as a tea or added to smoothies and juices. Depending on the desired benefit, the most effective way to consume ginger may vary.

- **Fresh Ginger**: Fresh ginger root can be grated, sliced, or minced and added to a variety of dishes, from stir-fries to soups and marinades. It can also be steeped in hot water to make a soothing tea. For nausea relief, chew on a small piece of fresh ginger.

- **Ginger Tea**: To make ginger tea, slice or grate 1-2 inches of fresh ginger and steep in boiling water for 10-15 minutes. Strain and sweeten with honey if desired. Ginger tea is an excellent remedy for digestive discomfort, colds, and sore throats.

- **Ginger Powder**: Ground ginger is a convenient way to add ginger's benefits to your diet. It can be used in baking, cooking, or added to smoothies and oatmeal. The powdered form is often used in ginger supplements and capsules for concentrated doses.

- **Ginger Supplements**: Ginger is available in supplement form, including capsules and extracts. A standard dosage for digestive or anti-inflammatory benefits is typically 500-1,000 mg of ginger extract, taken 2-3 times per day, but it's always important to follow the specific dosing guidelines on the product label.

- **Essential Oil**: Ginger essential oil can be used topically (when diluted with a carrier oil) to relieve muscle pain, reduce inflammation, or support digestion when massaged onto the abdomen. It can also be inhaled through aromatherapy to relieve nausea and improve focus.

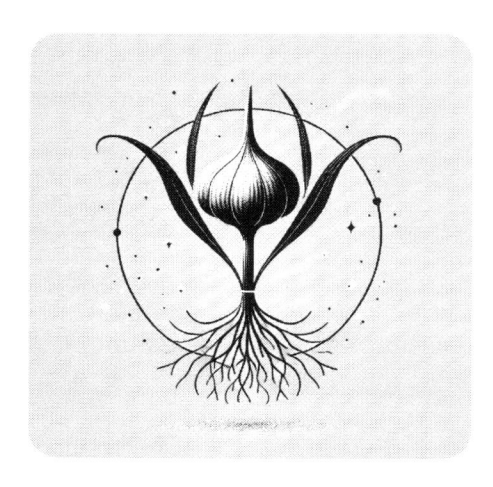

4. Garlic

Botanical Description:

Garlic (*Allium sativum*) is a hardy, perennial plant belonging to the *Amaryllidaceae* family, which also includes onions, leeks, and shallots. Native to Central Asia, garlic has been cultivated for over 5,000 years for both its culinary and medicinal uses. The plant grows up to 2-3 feet tall and produces long, flat leaves with a bulbous underground root, known as the garlic bulb. Each bulb is made up of several smaller cloves encased in a papery skin.

Garlic is easily recognized by its strong aroma and pungent flavor, which intensifies when the cloves are crushed or chopped. The primary compound responsible for garlic's distinctive smell and healing properties is **allicin**, a sulfur-containing compound that is released when garlic is crushed or chewed.

Healing Properties:

Garlic is revered for its potent medicinal qualities and has been used for centuries as a natural remedy to support cardiovascular health, boost the immune system, and prevent infections. Its rich content of bioactive compounds, particularly allicin, gives garlic a wide range of healing properties.

- **Supports Heart Health**: Garlic is well-known for its cardiovascular benefits, helping to lower blood pressure, reduce cholesterol levels, and improve circulation. Studies have shown that garlic can help lower LDL ("bad") cholesterol while raising HDL ("good") cholesterol. It also has mild blood-thinning properties, which help prevent blood clots and reduce the risk of heart disease and stroke.

- **Boosts Immune Function**: Garlic is a natural immune booster, stimulating the activity of white blood cells, which help the body fight infections. Regular consumption of garlic has been linked to a reduced risk of colds, flu, and other infections. Garlic's antiviral, antibacterial, and antifungal properties make it particularly effective in preventing and treating common infections.

- **Anti-Inflammatory and Antioxidant Effects**: Garlic contains antioxidants that help protect the body from oxidative damage and reduce inflammation, making it beneficial for individuals dealing with chronic inflammatory conditions such as arthritis. Allicin also has anti-inflammatory properties, which can help reduce swelling and pain.

- **Antimicrobial Properties**: Allicin, the key compound in garlic, is a potent antimicrobial agent. It has been shown to inhibit the growth of bacteria, viruses, and fungi. This makes garlic a natural remedy for treating infections like respiratory infections, fungal skin infections, and digestive issues caused by harmful bacteria.

- **Regulates Blood Sugar**: Garlic can help regulate blood sugar levels by improving insulin sensitivity. This makes it a useful dietary addition for individuals managing type 2 diabetes or prediabetes.

- **Detoxification**: Garlic contains sulfur compounds that support the detoxification process in the liver. By enhancing the production of detoxifying enzymes, garlic helps the body eliminate toxins and heavy metals.

Usage Guidelines:

Garlic is a versatile herb that can be used in its fresh, raw form or in cooked dishes, and it is also available in supplements, oils, and powders. The most potent health benefits come from consuming raw or lightly cooked garlic, as allicin is most active when garlic is fresh and unheated.

- **Raw Garlic**: For maximum medicinal benefits, garlic is best consumed raw. Crush or chop a clove of garlic and let it sit for 10 minutes to allow the allicin to fully activate. Raw garlic can be added to salad dressings, dips, or taken directly with water or honey to mask the strong taste.

- **Cooked Garlic**: While cooking reduces the potency of allicin, garlic still retains many of its benefits when cooked. Lightly sauté or roast garlic for use in a variety of dishes like soups, stir-fries, or roasted vegetables. Avoid overcooking garlic, as high heat for long periods can diminish its medicinal value.

- **Garlic Supplements**: Garlic supplements are available in capsule, powder, or oil form, often marketed as aged garlic extract or garlic oil. A standard daily dose ranges from 600-1,200 mg of garlic extract. Supplements may be a good option for individuals who cannot tolerate the strong taste or smell of fresh garlic.

- **Garlic Oil**: Garlic-infused oil can be used topically to treat fungal infections, ear infections, or to soothe skin conditions like acne. Garlic oil can also be consumed internally to support heart health.

- **Garlic Honey**: Garlic cloves can be infused in raw honey to create a natural remedy for colds, sore throats, and coughs. Simply peel a few garlic cloves and place them in a jar with honey. Let it sit for a few days, and take a spoonful daily to boost immunity.

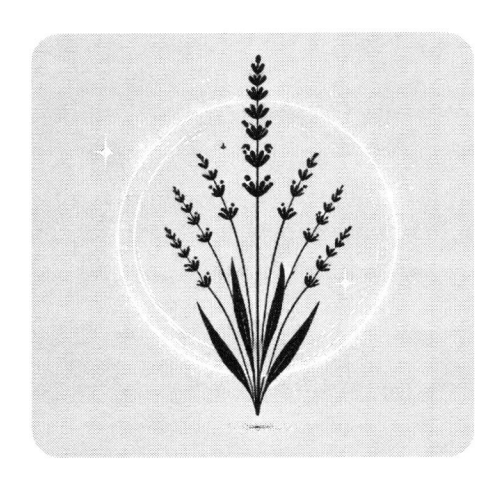

5. Lavender

Botanical Description:

Lavender (*Lavandula angustifolia*), a member of the *Lamiaceae* (mint) family, is a fragrant, perennial herb native to the Mediterranean region but now cultivated worldwide for its beauty, fragrance, and medicinal properties. Lavender grows in bushy clumps about 2-3 feet tall, producing slender stems with silvery-green leaves and vibrant purple or blue flowers. The plant thrives in sunny, well-drained soils and is known for its soothing, aromatic blossoms, which are harvested and dried for a variety of uses.

Lavender's essential oil, extracted from its flowers through steam distillation, contains powerful bioactive compounds such as **linalool** and **linalyl acetate**, which contribute to its calming, antimicrobial, and anti-inflammatory properties. This herb is one of the most versatile medicinal plants, commonly used in aromatherapy, skincare, and herbal remedies.

Healing Properties:

Lavender is cherished for its soothing and healing qualities, particularly for its ability to calm the nervous system, alleviate stress, and promote restful sleep. Its gentle, yet potent, effects make it a popular choice for treating a wide range of physical and emotional conditions.

- **Calms the Nervous System**: Lavender's most well-known benefit is its ability to reduce stress and anxiety. The herb works by affecting the parasympathetic nervous system, which helps the body relax. Inhaling lavender's scent or applying it topically can reduce anxiety, improve mood, and promote a sense of calm.

- **Promotes Sleep**: Lavender is commonly used to treat insomnia and other sleep disorders. Its mild sedative effect can help you fall asleep faster and improve the quality of sleep by reducing restlessness and promoting relaxation.

- **Anti-Inflammatory and Pain-Relieving**: Lavender's essential oil has anti-inflammatory and analgesic properties, making it useful for relieving headaches, muscle pain, and joint stiffness. It can also be used to soothe skin irritations, burns, and insect bites.

- **Antimicrobial and Antiseptic**: Lavender's antimicrobial properties make it a natural remedy for minor cuts, wounds, and infections. It has been traditionally used to clean wounds and prevent infection due to its antibacterial and antifungal effects.

- **Supports Skin Health**: Lavender oil is a popular ingredient in skincare products because of its ability to soothe irritated skin, reduce redness, and help heal conditions such as acne, eczema, and psoriasis. Its antimicrobial properties also make it effective in treating blemishes and promoting clearer skin.

- **Relieves Respiratory Symptoms**: Lavender has been used as an inhalant to relieve symptoms of colds, flu, asthma, and bronchitis. Its decongestant properties help to clear the airways, while its soothing effects calm coughs and reduce throat irritation.

Usage Guidelines:

Lavender can be used in various forms, including as an essential oil, dried herb, or tea. Its versatility allows it to be incorporated into daily life for both therapeutic and cosmetic purposes.

- **Essential Oil**: Lavender essential oil is one of the most widely used forms of lavender. It can be used for aromatherapy, applied topically, or added to bathwater for relaxation. To apply topically, dilute lavender essential oil with a carrier oil (such as coconut or almond oil) to avoid skin irritation. For stress relief, add a few drops of lavender oil to a diffuser or inhale directly from the bottle.

- **Lavender Tea**: Dried lavender flowers can be steeped in hot water to make a soothing tea that helps reduce stress and promotes restful sleep. To prepare, add 1-2 teaspoons of dried lavender buds to a cup of hot water, steep for 5-10 minutes, and strain. Lavender tea can be consumed before bed to promote relaxation.

- **Aromatherapy**: Lavender's scent can be used in a variety of ways to promote relaxation. Lavender-scented sachets can be placed under pillows, or a few drops of lavender oil can be sprinkled on bedding to enhance sleep quality. Lavender oil can also be added to bathwater for a calming soak.

- **Topical Applications**: Lavender oil can be used to treat minor burns, insect bites, and skin irritations by applying it diluted to the affected area. For headaches, lavender oil can be massaged into the temples, or a few drops can be added to a warm compress placed on the forehead.

- **Skincare**: Lavender-infused oils, creams, or balms can be applied to the skin to help with acne, eczema, or general skin inflammation. The antibacterial properties of lavender make it an excellent natural remedy for skin infections or blemishes.

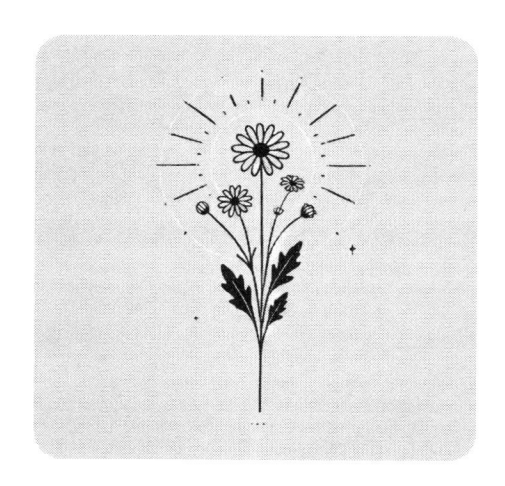

6. Chamomile

Botanical Description:

Chamomile refers to several daisy-like plants in the *Asteraceae* family, with the most common medicinal varieties being **German chamomile** (*Matricaria recutita*) and **Roman chamomile** (*Chamaemelum nobile*). Native to Europe and Western Asia, chamomile is now cultivated worldwide for its calming and healing properties. The plant typically grows about 1 to 2 feet tall, producing feathery leaves and small white flowers with bright yellow centers.

The flowers of the chamomile plant are the part most commonly used in herbal medicine, both fresh and dried. Chamomile flowers contain volatile oils, flavonoids, and other beneficial compounds like **apigenin**, which give it its distinctive soothing and anti-inflammatory properties.

Healing Properties:

Chamomile has been used for centuries as a gentle and effective remedy for a wide range of health issues, particularly for its calming, anti-inflammatory, and digestive benefits. It is especially well-known for promoting relaxation and sleep, but its uses extend far beyond that.

- **Promotes Relaxation and Sleep**: Chamomile is one of the most popular natural remedies for insomnia and anxiety. The herb contains **apigenin**, an antioxidant that binds to receptors in the brain and helps reduce anxiety, induce calmness, and promote sleep. Chamomile tea is often consumed before bed as a mild sedative to improve sleep quality and help with restlessness.

- **Anti-Inflammatory**: Chamomile has strong anti-inflammatory properties that make it useful for soothing various inflammatory conditions, including digestive issues, skin irritations, and joint pain. It helps reduce redness, swelling, and irritation, making it an excellent remedy for conditions like arthritis and eczema.

- **Aids Digestion**: Chamomile is frequently used to relieve digestive discomforts such as bloating, gas, and indigestion. Its calming effect on the digestive tract helps ease symptoms of irritable bowel syndrome (IBS), gastritis, and other gastrointestinal issues. Chamomile tea can also soothe stomach cramps and mild nausea.

- **Antispasmodic and Pain-Relieving**: Chamomile's antispasmodic properties help reduce muscle spasms and cramps, making it useful for menstrual pain, muscle aches, and tension headaches. It helps to relax smooth muscle tissue, easing discomfort and pain.

- **Supports Skin Health**: Chamomile's anti-inflammatory and antimicrobial properties make it effective for treating minor skin irritations, rashes, and wounds. It can soothe inflamed skin, reduce redness, and promote healing when applied topically. Chamomile is often found in skincare products for its ability to calm sensitive or irritated skin.

- **Antimicrobial**: Chamomile has mild antibacterial and antifungal properties, making it helpful for preventing and treating infections. It can be used as a natural remedy for minor cuts, scrapes, and sore throats caused by bacterial infections.

Usage Guidelines:

Chamomile can be used in a variety of forms, including as a tea, tincture, essential oil, or topical application. It is most commonly consumed as a tea, but its essential oil and extracts offer additional ways to incorporate its healing properties into your daily routine.

- **Chamomile Tea**: The most common way to use chamomile is in tea form, made from dried chamomile flowers. To prepare, steep 1-2 teaspoons of dried chamomile flowers in a cup of hot water for 5-10 minutes, then strain and enjoy. Chamomile tea is excellent for promoting relaxation, aiding digestion, and relieving stress. Drink 1-2 cups a day, especially before bed, to enhance sleep and calm the mind.

- **Tincture or Extract**: Chamomile is available in concentrated liquid extracts or tinctures. These can be taken orally to relieve stress, promote sleep, or improve digestion. The standard dosage for chamomile tincture is usually 30-40 drops in water or juice, taken 1-3 times per day, depending on the condition being treated.

- **Chamomile Essential Oil**: Chamomile essential oil can be used in aromatherapy or applied topically (when diluted) to soothe skin irritations or promote relaxation. Add a few drops of chamomile essential oil to a diffuser to reduce stress and create a calming environment, or dilute with a carrier oil and apply to the skin for pain relief or to treat skin conditions.

- **Topical Applications**: Chamomile can be used as a compress or in creams to treat skin irritations such as eczema, rashes, or wounds. To make a chamomile compress, steep a strong chamomile tea and soak a cloth in the tea before applying it to the affected area for 10-15 minutes.

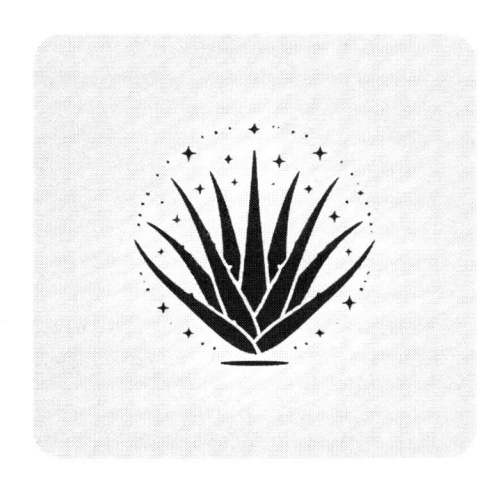

7. Aloe Vera

Botanical Description:

Aloe vera (*Aloe barbadensis miller*) is a succulent plant belonging to the *Asphodelaceae* family, native to the Arabian Peninsula but now cultivated worldwide for its medicinal and cosmetic uses. Aloe vera grows in arid, tropical climates and is known for its thick, fleshy, greenish-gray leaves that store a translucent gel. This gel is rich in bioactive compounds and is used for a variety of health and skincare purposes.

The leaves of the aloe vera plant grow from the base in a rosette pattern and can reach lengths of 12 to 19 inches. The plant also produces yellow tubular flowers on tall spikes, though it is the gel inside the leaves that holds the majority of its healing properties. Aloe vera gel is composed of 99% water, but it also contains essential vitamins, minerals, enzymes, amino acids, and antioxidants, making it a potent natural remedy for both internal and external use.

Healing Properties:

Aloe vera is one of the most versatile and widely used medicinal plants, with a long history of use in treating various skin conditions, promoting healing, and supporting overall health. The plant's soothing, anti-inflammatory, and antimicrobial properties make it effective for treating burns, wounds, and skin irritations, while its digestive benefits have earned it a reputation as a remedy for gut health.

- **Soothes Burns and Skin Irritations**: Aloe vera is most famous for its ability to soothe and heal burns, including sunburns. Its cooling gel provides immediate relief from heat and inflammation, while its compounds help accelerate the healing process of minor burns and skin injuries. Aloe also helps relieve itching and irritation caused by eczema, psoriasis, and rashes.

- **Promotes Wound Healing**: Aloe vera has powerful skin-repairing properties. It stimulates fibroblasts, the cells responsible for wound healing, which helps close wounds faster. Aloe also increases collagen production, aiding in the healing of cuts, scrapes, and surgical wounds.

- **Hydrates and Nourishes the Skin**: Aloe vera gel is deeply moisturizing, making it an ideal natural remedy for dry or sensitive skin. It helps lock in moisture without clogging pores, making it suitable for all skin types, including acne-prone skin. Its rich nutrient content, including vitamins C and E, supports skin regeneration and elasticity.

- **Anti-Inflammatory and Antimicrobial**: Aloe vera contains compounds such as **aloins** and **polysaccharides** that reduce inflammation and protect against infection. Its antimicrobial effects make it useful for treating acne, fungal infections, and minor bacterial infections.

- **Supports Digestive Health**: Taken internally, aloe vera juice has been traditionally used to soothe and heal the digestive tract. It can relieve symptoms of irritable bowel syndrome (IBS), acid reflux, and ulcers by reducing inflammation and promoting healthy digestion. Aloe vera also has mild laxative properties that can help alleviate constipation.

- **Boosts Immune Function**: Aloe vera contains antioxidants, including vitamins A, C, and E, that help combat oxidative stress and support the immune system. The plant's natural compounds help modulate immune function, making it beneficial for overall health.

Usage Guidelines:

Aloe vera can be used topically or taken internally, depending on the desired benefit. Fresh aloe gel is the most potent form, but commercially prepared aloe vera gels, creams, and juices are also widely available. When using aloe vera internally, be sure to choose products labeled for internal use, as some formulations are only intended for topical application.

- **Topical Use**: To use aloe vera topically, simply cut an aloe vera leaf and scoop out the clear gel. Apply the gel directly to burns, wounds, or irritated skin. Aloe vera can be applied multiple times per day to promote healing and reduce inflammation. It is particularly effective for treating sunburns, minor cuts, insect bites, and dry skin.

- **Aloe Vera Gel**: Commercial aloe vera gels are available for topical use and often include additional ingredients to enhance their moisturizing or healing effects. Choose a product with a high concentration of pure aloe and minimal additives for best results.

- **Aloe Vera Juice**: Aloe vera juice is taken internally to support digestive health, relieve constipation, and reduce inflammation. The recommended dosage is generally 1-2 tablespoons of aloe vera juice per day, mixed with water or juice. Start with a small amount to gauge your body's response, as aloe's laxative properties can affect some individuals more strongly than others.

- **Aloe Vera Supplements**: Aloe vera is also available in capsule or tablet form, typically used to support digestive health or boost immune function. Follow the dosage recommendations on the product label.

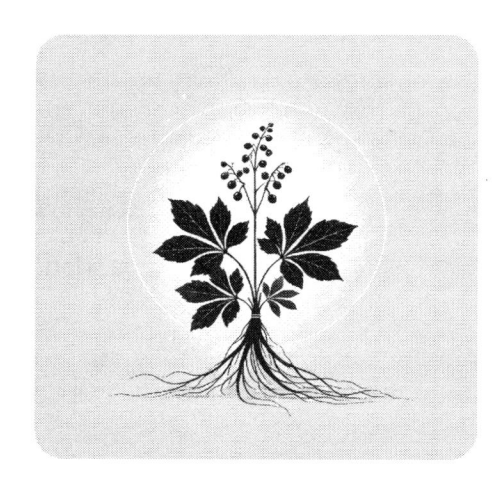

8. Ginseng

Botanical Description:

Ginseng refers to a group of slow-growing perennial plants with fleshy roots that belong to the *Araliaceae* family. The two most common and widely studied types are **Asian ginseng** (*Panax ginseng*), native to Korea and China, and **American ginseng** (*Panax quinquefolius*), native to North America. The name *Panax* means "all-healing," reflecting ginseng's revered status in traditional medicine systems for its broad range of health benefits.

Ginseng plants are known for their forked, fleshy roots, long stalks, and green leaves that grow in a circular pattern. The root is the part used medicinally, either fresh or dried. Ginseng roots typically have a human-like shape, which has contributed to its symbolic and medicinal value in ancient cultures. The active compounds in ginseng are called **ginsenosides** (or **panaxosides**), which are responsible for many of its health-promoting properties.

Healing Properties:

Ginseng is considered one of the most potent adaptogens, meaning it helps the body adapt to stress and restore balance. It is valued for its ability to enhance energy, improve cognitive function, and support overall well-being. Ginseng's versatile health benefits have made it a staple in both traditional Chinese medicine (TCM) and Western herbal medicine.

- **Boosts Energy and Reduces Fatigue**: Ginseng is widely known for its energy-boosting effects. It helps increase physical and mental endurance, making it a popular remedy for combating fatigue, especially in individuals experiencing chronic fatigue or those recovering from illness. It also supports the adrenal glands, helping to regulate the body's stress response.

- **Improves Cognitive Function**: Ginseng enhances mental clarity, focus, and memory by increasing blood circulation to the brain and improving neurotransmitter function. It is often used to boost concentration and cognitive performance, making it beneficial for students, professionals, or older adults experiencing age-related cognitive decline.

- **Supports Immune Function**: Ginseng helps modulate the immune system, enhancing the body's ability to fight infections and improve overall immune function. Studies have shown that it can reduce the frequency and severity of colds and flu by stimulating the production of white blood cells.

- **Adaptogen for Stress**: As an adaptogen, ginseng helps the body cope with both physical and emotional stress. It balances cortisol levels, reducing the impact of stress on the body, and supports overall emotional and physical resilience.

- **Anti-Inflammatory**: Ginseng contains powerful anti-inflammatory compounds, making it useful for reducing inflammation in the body. Its antioxidant effects also help protect cells from damage caused by oxidative stress, which is linked to aging and chronic diseases.

- **Supports Sexual Health**: Ginseng has traditionally been used as a natural remedy for improving libido and sexual performance in both men and women. In men, it can help improve erectile function by increasing nitric oxide production, which enhances blood flow. In women, ginseng may help balance hormones and increase energy levels, thereby improving sexual vitality.

Usage Guidelines:

Ginseng can be consumed in various forms, including capsules, powders, teas, tinctures, and extracts. Depending on the intended use, ginseng can be taken daily to support energy and well-being or during periods of stress or fatigue.

- **Ginseng Tea**: To make ginseng tea, use 1-2 grams of dried ginseng root (or a teaspoon of ginseng powder) and steep it in hot water for about 10-15 minutes. You can also add honey or lemon for flavor. Ginseng tea is a simple way to boost energy and focus, especially when consumed in the morning or early afternoon.

- **Ginseng Capsules or Tablets**: Ginseng is commonly available in capsule or tablet form for daily supplementation. Standard dosages for general well-being range from 200-400 mg per day of ginseng extract, though higher doses may be used for specific conditions. It is often recommended to take ginseng with food to avoid potential stomach upset.

- **Ginseng Extracts and Tinctures**: Liquid ginseng extracts or tinctures provide a concentrated form of the herb and can be taken in small doses. A typical dose is 1-2 ml of ginseng extract, taken up to 3 times per day, depending on the product and intended use. These extracts can be added to water, tea, or juice for easier consumption.

- **Ginseng Powder**: Ginseng powder can be added to smoothies, soups, or teas for an easy way to incorporate the herb into your diet. The recommended dose of powdered ginseng is typically 1-2 grams per day.

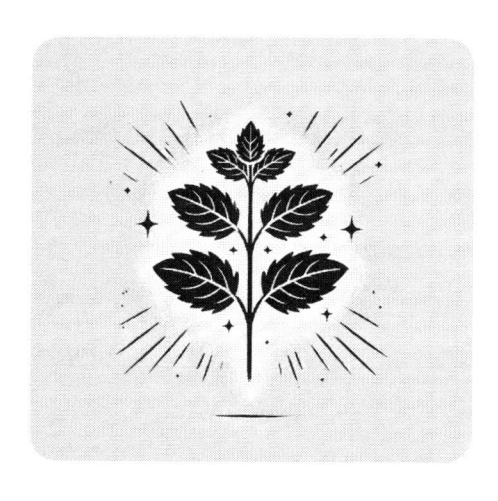

9. Peppermint

Botanical Description:

- **Family:** Lamiaceae (Mint family)
- **Appearance:** Peppermint is a perennial herb that typically grows to about 30-90 cm (12-36 inches) tall. It has dark green leaves with reddish veins and stems that are usually purple-tinged. The leaves are aromatic, smooth, and ovate with serrated edges.
- **Flowers:** The plant produces small, pale purple to violet flowers that bloom in spikes.
- **Habitat:** Peppermint grows best in moist, shaded locations and is often cultivated in herb gardens. It can also grow in wild, temperate areas.

Healing Properties:

- **Digestive Aid:** Peppermint is commonly used to alleviate indigestion, bloating, and gas. Its antispasmodic properties help relax the muscles of the digestive tract.
- **Relief from Irritable Bowel Syndrome (IBS):** Peppermint oil capsules are often recommended for managing symptoms of IBS, such as cramping and abdominal pain.
- **Respiratory Support:** The menthol in peppermint acts as a natural decongestant, making it useful for relieving symptoms of colds, coughs, and sinus congestion.
- **Pain Relief:** Peppermint oil can be applied topically to relieve headaches, muscle pain, and joint discomfort due to its cooling and anti-inflammatory properties.
- **Antimicrobial:** Peppermint has antimicrobial and antifungal properties, making it useful in oral care products to freshen breath and fight infections.
- **Mental Clarity and Focus:** Inhaling peppermint essential oil or using it in aromatherapy can help improve focus, reduce mental fatigue, and enhance alertness.

Usage Guidelines:

- **Tea:** Peppermint tea is commonly brewed to aid digestion, soothe upset stomachs, and relieve headaches. Steep 1-2 teaspoons of dried leaves in hot water for 5-10 minutes.

- **Essential Oil:** Peppermint essential oil can be used for aromatherapy or applied topically (diluted with a carrier oil) to relieve pain or headaches. A few drops can be inhaled or diffused for mental clarity.

- **Capsules:** Peppermint oil capsules are often taken to alleviate digestive issues, such as IBS, but should be enteric-coated to prevent irritation of the stomach lining.

- **Topical Use:** For muscle or joint pain, dilute peppermint oil with a carrier oil (like coconut or jojoba) and massage into the affected area.

- **Inhalation:** For sinus or respiratory issues, inhaling the vapors of peppermint essential oil (using a steam bowl or diffuser) can help clear nasal passages.

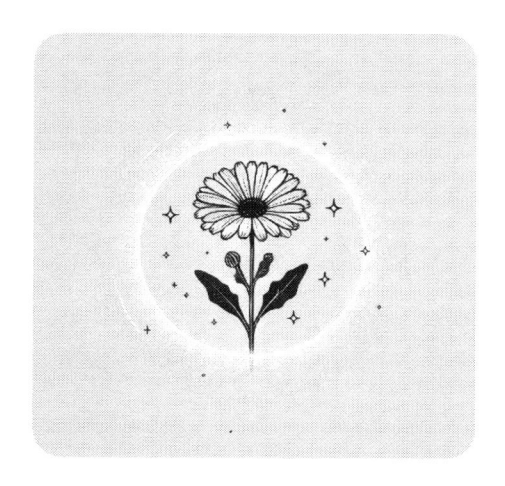

10. Calendula

Botanical Description:

- **Family:** Asteraceae (Daisy family)

- **Appearance:** Calendula, also known as pot marigold, is a hardy annual plant that grows between 30-60 cm (12-24 inches) tall. It has bright green, lance-shaped leaves and produces vivid yellow or orange flowers.

- **Flowers:** The flowers are the most notable part of the plant, featuring a daisy-like appearance with multiple layers of petals. These flowers are edible and used in herbal preparations.

- **Habitat:** Native to the Mediterranean region, calendula thrives in well-drained, moderately rich soil and full sunlight. It is commonly grown in gardens and is often cultivated for its medicinal flowers.

Healing Properties:

- **Wound Healing:** Calendula is widely recognized for its ability to speed up the healing of wounds, cuts, and minor burns due to its anti-inflammatory and antimicrobial properties. It helps promote tissue regeneration.

- **Skin Care:** Calendula is a popular remedy for skin conditions such as eczema, dermatitis, rashes, and insect bites. It soothes irritated skin, reduces redness, and promotes hydration, making it useful in skincare products for sensitive or dry skin.

- **Anti-Inflammatory:** It has strong anti-inflammatory properties, making it useful for reducing swelling and inflammation, both externally (as a cream or salve) and internally (as tea or tincture).

- **Antiseptic and Antimicrobial:** Calendula's antimicrobial effects help fight infections in minor wounds, cuts, and scrapes, preventing bacterial growth.

- **Oral Health:** Calendula can be used in mouthwashes or gargles to reduce inflammation in the mouth and throat, helping with conditions like gingivitis and sore throats.

- **Antifungal:** Calendula has been shown to have antifungal properties, making it beneficial in treating fungal infections such as athlete's foot or ringworm.

Usage Guidelines:

- **Tea:** Calendula tea can be made by steeping 1-2 teaspoons of dried calendula flowers in hot water for 10 minutes. It is often used for its soothing effects on the digestive tract or to relieve inflammation in the mouth and throat.

- **Topical Application:** Calendula is commonly used in ointments, creams, and salves for skin irritations, wounds, rashes, and burns. It can be applied directly to the affected area to promote healing and reduce inflammation.

- **Infused Oil:** Calendula flowers can be infused in oil (such as olive or almond oil) to create a soothing oil that is applied topically for dry, chapped, or irritated skin. This infused oil is often used as a base for making salves or creams.

- **Tincture:** Calendula tincture can be used internally for its anti-inflammatory and antiseptic properties or diluted for topical use to clean wounds.

- **Compress:** Calendula flowers can be made into a compress by soaking them in warm water, which can then be applied to skin irritations, wounds, or sore muscles.

170. Bonus Ch. 10 - The Top 10 Healing Plants - Detailed Profiles

Top 10 Most Used Medicinal Herbs and Their Popularity

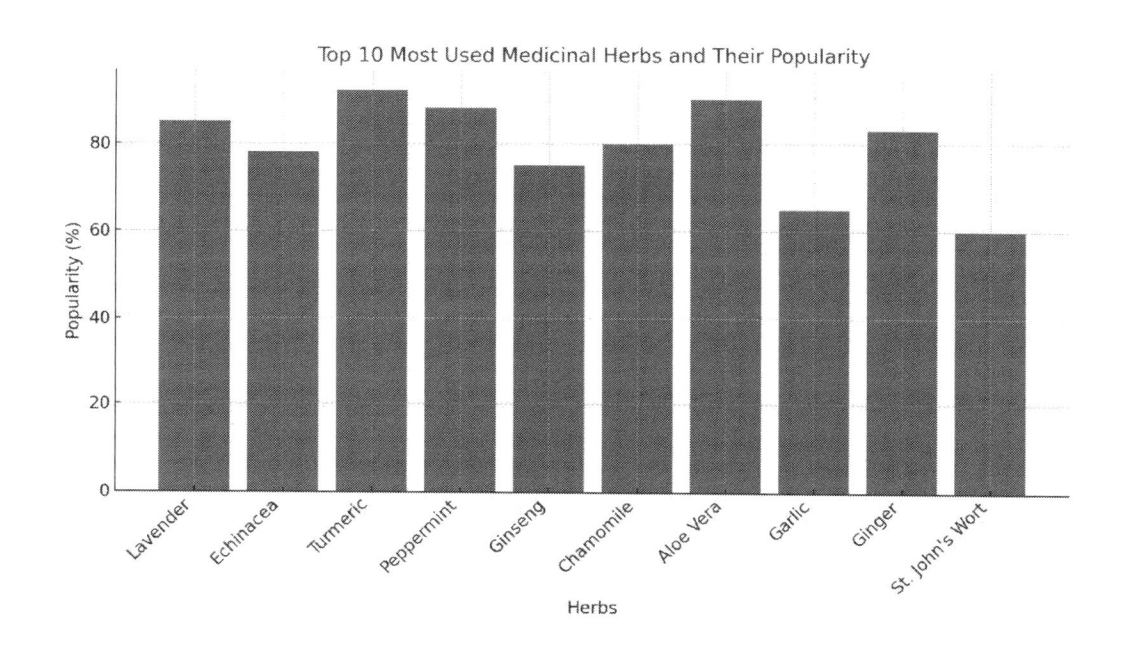

Here is the chart showing the 10 most commonly used medicinal herbs and their popularity, represented as a percentage. Herbs like turmeric, lavender, and aloe vera are among the most popular, used for a variety of medicinal applications.

Conclusion

As we conclude this journey through *The Lost Bible of Natural Herbal Remedies*, it's clear that nature has always been a profound source of healing. Across millennia, ancient civilizations have turned to the earth's flora to treat illnesses, enhance vitality, and promote overall well-being. These time-tested recipes not only highlight the remarkable medicinal properties of plants but also connect us to a deep, ancestral wisdom that still holds relevance in our modern world.

In an age where synthetic medicines often dominate healthcare, there is a growing appreciation for holistic approaches that consider the body, mind, and spirit as an interconnected whole. By rediscovering the power of these natural remedies, we tap into a legacy of healing that prioritizes balance, prevention, and respect for the body's innate capacity to heal itself.

As you explore the 100+ ancient healing recipes shared in this book, remember that natural remedies, while powerful, require mindful application and respect. The key to their effectiveness lies not just in the plants themselves but in the wisdom of how and when to use them. Whether you seek relief from common ailments, wish to boost your vitality, or simply want to integrate nature's gifts into your daily life, these herbal recipes offer a versatile toolkit for health and wellness.

Ultimately, this book is more than just an encyclopedia of herbal remedies – it's an invitation to reconnect with the earth, to honor the wisdom of our ancestors, and to cultivate a life of holistic health. May the knowledge contained within these pages empower you to live with greater harmony, resilience, and appreciation for the natural world.

As you continue your journey, may you find healing, balance, and well-being through the age-old art of herbal medicine. The wisdom of the past is now in your hands, ready to be integrated into the present, and carried forward into the future.

172. Regards

Regards

Dear Reader,

Thank you for taking the time to read this book and for reaching its conclusion.

Your commitment means more to me than words can express, as it brings life to my work, and I am deeply grateful to you.

If this reading has satisfied and helped you, I would be truly appreciative if you could take a moment to leave a review. Such feedback is invaluable – it helps other readers discover this work and provides me with inspiration to continue improving as a writer.

Thank you with all my heart.

Call to action **.173**

Scan the QR to access the free bonus: audiobook!

Leave a review ▶

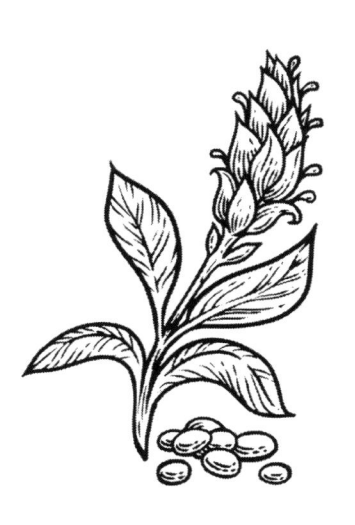

Made in the USA
Monee, IL
02 March 2025